fat like us

fat like us

Jean Renfro Anspaugh

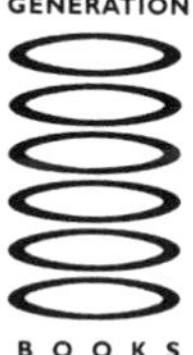

An imprint of Windows on History Press, Inc.
Durham, North Carolina

GENERATION

BOOKS

Published by Generation Books
604 Brookwood Drive
Durham, NC 27707
phone/fax 919.489.7759

5 4 3 2 1

Design and composition by Chris Crochetière,
B. Williams & Associates, Durham, North Carolina

Generation Books ISBN 0-9654499-5-5

This is a work of creative nonfiction. The persons described in this work, except where cited, are merely composites and do not pertain to any person living or deceased. All names, locations, professions, and ages have been changed.

Visit Generation Books online at
www.generationbooks.com
Fat Like Us online at
www.fatlikeus.com

Library of Congress Cataloging-in-Publication Data
Anspaugh, Jean Renfro, 1953–
Fat like us / Jean Renfro Anspaugh.
p. cm.
Includes bibliographical references.
ISBN 0-9654499-5-5
1. Weight loss—North Carolina—Durham.
2. Obesity—Social aspects—United States. I. Title.
RM222.2 .A545 2001
616.3'98'00973—dc21 2001040360

To the memory of Clara

contents

introduction

Diet Culture

How I Came to Meet My Own Kind

One evening I was sitting on the patio of my house in Sacramento listening to my mother go on and on about what I should do with my future and how I had wasted my endless opportunities. I turned and saw her as a disembodied head. Her voice sounded as though she was speaking in a tunnel. The words she mouthed got lost in the night sounds of crickets and birds and in the sounds of cars honking on the highway in the distance. The honking turned into a siren screaming and went on and on. I realized it wasn't a police car or an ambulance, but me. My mother had vanished into the house, my neighbors' yard lights were switched on, and I was sitting on the concrete floor of my patio, still screaming. The folding lounge chair I was sitting on had collapsed under my immense weight. Two weeks later, I was in Durham, North Carolina—a patient on the Rice Diet and neophyte in Ricer culture.

A sign on Highway I-85 once proclaimed WELCOME TO DURHAM—DIET CAPITAL OF THE WORLD. For me and thousands of people like me, this sign symbolized a threshold: a gateway to a new and better life. We come to North Carolina hoping to obtain a thin body and all that it grants. Buddy Hackett, Wendy Wasserstein, Dom DeLuise, Marilyn Horne, Mario Puzo, James Coco, talk show hosts, Supreme

Court justices, television sitcom stars, NFL players, rappers, and even Elvis all raved about their monumental weight losses in Durham. Ordinary dieters who come to Durham fat and return home thin are walking testimonies to the power of dieting in Durham. Our success stories travel through the fat underground like talismans passed from one fat person to another.

In cities across America we had joined diet programs such as Weight Watchers, Diet Center, Jenny Craig, Physicians Weight Loss Center, and Nutri/System. Every hospital in any medium-sized town has an in-house medical fast program such as Optifast or Medifast as well as exercise and behavior-modification classes. In community centers and churches, people gather at Overeaters Anonymous, Foodaholics Anonymous, TOPS (Take Off Pounds Sensibly), Positive Weigh meetings, and Weigh Down workshops. Each day another bestseller hits bookstores hailing a faster and better way to take off unwanted pounds and find inner healing, spiritual peace, and true health. Talk show hosts interview the rich and famous about their weight-loss regimens; even the hosts themselves reveal their personal struggles with weight. With the vast extent of the available information on diet and weight control and all the medical attention given to them, why would anyone leave home and venture forth to Durham? As one veteran dieter puts it, "Every fat person on earth knows in the back of his mind that Durham exists: mecca of the dieters. When all else fails, go to Durham."[1]

I had known about Durham all my life. I had always known about the Rice Diet. I knew it was where the fattest of the fat went for the last battle with their weight. Failures of other dieting programs, the morbidly obese, end up in Durham to confront their escalating weight and health problems. In the front room of the Rice House, they were weighed on one of two sets of scales: either the one for those people weighing under three hundred pounds or the one for those weighing more. Rumor had it that some dieters must be weighed on truck scales, and some have topped the twelve-hundred-pound mark. At 120 pounds overweight, I was about average for a new dieter in Durham.

I knew I was in the right place. I chose the Kempner Rice Diet from other nationally known diet programs because it is the oldest diet program in America. It is also the most rigorous. Due to its sheer longevity and the success stories of its participants, the Rice Diet seemed like the best program for me. The Rice Diet is for hard-core do-or-die dieters. It's the Marines of the diet programs. Long-term dieter Kenneth Meyer asserted, "It is just like boot camp. Sooner or later the food catches up with you and you got to go to Durham. It's where we must come to pay for our sins."[2] I wanted a diet that was hard, I wanted it to be hard and fast and brutal, and if it didn't cure me, I wanted it to kill me. Once in Durham, I met a community of dieters who felt as I did and who had, in fact, shared almost exactly the same life experiences that I had. It was a revelation to me.

Obesity cuts across race, class, gender, and nationality. Though diverse, we Ricers were identified by our body fat, and that identity superseded any personal distinctions we might have brought with us to Durham. The weight that once separated us from the dominant society now united us in diet culture.

We all were overweight and had been on and off diets throughout our lives. We might have had periods of thinness that sometimes lasted for several years, but we had always returned to an obese state. We had been on many diet and exercise programs. Most of us had started our dieting lives with Weight Watchers. Our dieting attempts could have served as a history of the popular theories of American medicine. Dieters in my age category had tried Dexatrim, coffee, amphetamines, and phenobarbital in the early 1960s. In the early 1970s we followed up with shots of human chorionic gonadotropin (HCG) along with a five-hundred-calorie-a-day diet, papaya, and garlic pills, and in the 1990s we tried fenfluramine as the cure for obesity and depression and dexfenfluramine for diet adherence. The millennium brought us prescription fat blockers.

We counted calories, fat grams, and carbohydrates, weighed and measured all of our food and liquid, ate within the zone, ate mindfully and with serenity. We were applauded when we lost a pound at Weight Watchers meetings; we were accepted as fellow sufferers at Overeaters Anonymous meetings; we admitted we were disobedient children of God at Weigh Down workshops; we toted our Jenny Craig lunches, our Nutri/System complete meals, our Physicians Weight Loss protein drinks, and our Diet Center supplements wherever we went; we journaled our feelings to reveal any unmet need that might have caused us to overeat.

The oldest group of dieters among us remembered taking thyroid pills and insecticide-based drugs to curb hunger. Their flesh had been bound in rubber suits to melt off fat. Their wobbly thighs had been pummeled by passive exercise machines. They had eaten protein lunches and abstained from consuming carbohydrates. A generation later, their sons and daughters eschewed fat and consumed carbohydrates as the key to weight loss. They shook their loose booties at high-intensity step aerobics and jazzercize classes. Coming full circle, their children now eat protein just like their grandparents did so long ago. The youngest Ricers do kickboxing and power yoga and have suffered a range of eating disorders from bulimia to anorexia. They have endured liposuction and gastric surgery on their quest for thinness.

We all had a history of trying popular diets, and our bodies, hearts, and minds still carried the effects of those years of struggle and accumulated dieting experience. Our bodies were witnesses to our diet failures. Each of us had met our every need and emotion with the great comforter—food. We agreed that overeating was acceptable and even encouraged in our society by all-you-can-eat buffets, super-sized fast food meals, twenty-ounce cokes, and king-size candy bars. However, we also knew gaining weight and getting fat from all that consumption was not acceptable. To us, food had become a complex source of nourishment and conflict. We used food and overeating as the coping mechanisms that helped us get through the hard parts of life.

Many of us had developed elaborate systems to obtain excess food. One dieter informed me that she used to go to the bakery of a local supermarket and explain to the bored clerk that she had to have a large amount of baked goods because she was a nurse's aide in a house of elderly women. She would detail the illness of each imaginary woman, explaining how a particular pastry was a dying request from one of them. Another dieter told me that he would often go into a restaurant and order two meals, telling the waitress that he was waiting for a friend. He'd tote the excess food away in a carry-out bag, only to eat it in the car. Some dieters would shop at food warehouses and stock up on chips, soda, and frozen cakes so they could be prepared just in case forty hungry people showed up at their house. They ended up eating the food themselves. I would go through the cafeteria line at work, and as the food piled up I would tell the cashier that I was purchasing food for fellow workers. I would go to the ladies' room and eat just a bite out of each pile of food, some mashed potatoes here, a bite of fried chicken there, a spoonful of pudding. Then I would toss the rest into the trash can and return to my office.

Food was the way to calm the waters of our angry lives. Female dieters used chocolate and ice cream as drugs. Dieters told of unconscious eating events in which they consumed large amounts of comfort food without even knowing it. One dieter remembered waking up one morning surrounded by empty pint-sized Häagen-Dazs coffee ice cream cartons. She had no idea how they had appeared in her bedroom, or if she had actually eaten the ice cream. Her story was a familiar one. All of us in diet culture self-medicate with food. Excess food does help us cope, but ultimately our source of temporary comfort becomes the core of chronic pain.

We had successful lives as bankers, lawyers, doctors, and businesspeople. Some of us had suffered great tragedy and pain, and brought a history of physical and sexual abuse with us to Durham. Many of the women had been raped during adolescence. We had responded to the violence perpetrated against us by building a defensive wall of flesh. We internalized the horror, spoke rarely of it, and instead let our bodies say what we were unable to voice.

The men among us externalized their pain, bringing to Durham a free-floating rage at the injustice of their plight and the weakness of their bodies. They saw their excessive weight as a personal and professional threat. They believed that they were at war with their bodies and would someday win that war. We women, on the other hand, felt that our fat was a personal sin that we carried publicly, like a scarlet letter, for all the world to see and judge. We embraced the weight struggle, interpreting our failures as moral ones and our successes as wonderful blessings that occurred randomly and only to the chosen few.

Perversely, we saw ourselves not only as the punished, but as the chosen. We believed that because of the way our weight had shaped us and our experiences, we had an abundance of spirit as well as flesh. We prided ourselves on our adaptability and our success at negotiating our bodies through the hostile territory of the dominant thin culture. We believed we could survive anything because we had developed skills for getting by. We thought of ourselves as passionate people with huge appetites for all that life had to offer: food, sex, laughter, and pain.

In Durham, in a community of dieters, I was with my own kind. I was no longer living a single, isolated life, but instead was part of a communal experience. For the first time, I felt at home and at peace with myself and my body. I was no longer the fattest person in a room, I was just normal. I didn't have to be the smartest or funniest, I could just be me. It is the number of dieters present that makes Durham so powerful for weight loss and personal transformation.

When we sat around the front porch of the Rice House and talked after meals, conversations that started out with pleasant comments on the weather or enthusiasm about another pound lost turned to litanies of life experiences and testimonies to the power of dieting and the redemptive, creative, and transformative value of long-sought thinness. Our conversations became oral histories of the fat life experience as well as critiques of our lifelong dieting attempts. Listening to other dieters share their testimonies, I learned that my life—with all its pain and failure, and resulting disappointment and shame—was not unique. We Ricers were representative of every popular diet in America and carried a diet wisdom and experience as well as a repertoire of dieting strategies and techniques. We know what it means to be fat, how to lose weight, and how to cope with regain. These practices of dieting can be viewed as rituals of weight loss and may be universally applied to all weight loss attempts. We speak to a *culture* of dieting—separate from and parallel to the dominant one, what mainstream white America finds attractive. It is the dominant image that tells us to be thin and depicts popular body types on the covers of magazines and in the movies.

A Culture Defined

Anthropologists believe that a culture is composed of the shared knowledge, beliefs, arts, morals, laws, customs, language, and religion of a particular group of people. Culture is learned and shared through behavior and oral traditions. To be truly powerful, a culture must distinguish itself from the others around it and form its own community. Through isolation, the community becomes homogeneous and solidifies its core values, which results in a group identity or belief system. This is especially true of disenfranchised minority groups. Obese individuals are ostracized from the main culture and constitute such a group. In the United States today, dieting is a separate culture. It has its own values, language, and modes of behavior, which are passed on orally through dieters' personal narrative experiences. This shared understanding guides behavior and informs dieters of the meaning of diet culture. Nowhere is this culture more visible or bonded more closely together than in Durham.

We members of diet culture value the same ideals that thin culture does, but not to the same extent. Though Western society prizes weight loss and thinness, to a dieter thinness is a relative concept. A person can be thought of as thin in Durham but fat anywhere else. Someone who weighs two hundred pounds looks small compared to those who weigh twice that much. At home that same two-hundred-pound person may feel fat and be regarded as such by others.

As diet culture's capital, Durham is unique because it is the only place in America where the obese can feel truly normal and at ease. We can move through our daily lives with confidence and grace. What appears abnormal and perhaps obscene to the rest of America is ordinary here. We can walk around the streets of Durham in shorts and tank tops—loose flesh flapping in the summer breeze—and not provoke one hand gesture or shout of indignation from passing cars. Only in Durham can a man who is 150 pounds overweight and far past his prime find himself surrounded by a bevy of beauties—large ones, yes, but beauties nevertheless, and young and eager for attention. Only in Durham can a 190-pound woman be considered a sex goddess and feel glorious in an XL bikini purchased from one of the many specialty stores that cater to the large. She can often be found poolside at Duke Towers, the apartment complex frequented by dieters, known to locals as the Whale Watch.

When I arrived in Durham at the age of thirty-four, with twenty-six years of dieting history behind me, I wasn't thinking about what constitutes culture. All I knew was that I was finally in the city devoted to dieters and weight loss, and for the first time in my life I would be able to focus on my life's preoccupation—obesity—without the distractions of job, school, family, or well-meaning friends. In Durham, I would find the magical cure that would relieve me of my excess weight. I would emerge, butterfly-like, from layers and layers of fat into a beautifully thin body and a much better life.

Giving Voice to My Culture

I lost seventy pounds in four months on the Rice Diet. Due to the program's expense, I soon ran out of money. Rather than leave Durham before I reached goal weight, I convinced the doctors at Duke to give me a job and pay me with reduced medical fees rather than a salary. My job was to help develop a database and profile of dieting patients. The doctors' focus was biomedical. They were interested in the statistical compilation of blood chemistries and the effect rice, fruit, and a very low calorie diet had on such chemistries. My interest, however, was cultural. Who were all these people, and why did we end up on diets in Durham? I wanted to know each patient's life story. As an employee of the Kempner Rice Clinic, I got both the reduced medical fees I needed to continue the program and access to almost fifty years of diet history. Also, through interacting with the doctors daily, I saw how they viewed their role in diet culture, which was a very different perspective from a dieter's.

I still didn't have any money to pay for meals, so I convinced the principal owner of the Rice House to hire me as a waitress and dishwasher and pay me with food rather than a salary. As a waitress at the Rice House, I received the meals that I needed as part of the program. I was also able to interact with patients, staff, and owners and see how they thought of their roles in the diet community. After a one-hundred-pound weight loss, I left the Rice Diet to attend the University of North Carolina at Chapel Hill and obtain a master's degree in folklore.

For a class project in an introduction to folklore course, I decided to collect dieters' life stories. I advertised in local newspapers, and I put up posters and announcements in coffee shops and on telephone poles. I walked around the streets of Durham with a miniature tape recorder stuck to my fanny pack. I walked from the Dieter's trek (beginning at the corner of Trinity Avenue and Mangum Street) to Ninth Street Bakery (now Elmo's Diner) for coffee and conversation with some burned-out bakery boys, and back up to Cardiac Hill for the final exhausting climb to the Rice House. I danced my nights away at the Crisco Disco, and snuck away with members of the Five Hundred Club to the delights and pleasures of Sin City for secret forbidden evenings. (These are dieters'— and specifically Ricers'—terms. I've provided a glossary of Ricer expressions at the end of this book.) The morning after those nights of indulgence, I followed in dieters' footsteps as they looked for a diuretic cure to purge their bodies of telltale sodium intake before the Rice House's morning ritual of weigh-in.

I could never leave behind the events I had witnessed and the stories I had heard in Durham. In school I studied different cultures and ethnic groups and wondered why nobody applied these concepts to dieters. As a folklorist, I was interested in the correspondence between culture and body image and how the two met at a sacred crossroads in Durham, a place where wishes were granted for a price. I was particularly interested in dieters' stories as vehicles for expressing and learning the values of diet culture. I was hoping to find the key to my struggle with obesity. Some authorities predict that ninety-five percent of the people who actually manage to lose weight will regain it within five years. I was determined to be in the lucky five percent, but I had no idea how to go about it. I thought that by researching patient case histories and talking to successful as well as failed dieters, I might be able to discern the secret of weight loss and maintenance.

I tried to find out why there was so little research on or even interest in dieters as a separate culture. Surely in America, where some studies suggest that half of the adult population is considered overweight and where we spend billions of dollars each year trying to get thin, I would be able to find some kind of report on who dieters really are. Yet experts in the weight-loss field had no advice for me. All I could find were diet books: books on how to lose weight, nothing on dieters themselves.

Why would a folklorist write about dieters? Folklorists have typically studied Shakers and Cajuns, or quilters and potters, or blues singers and whirligig makers, but not dieters. Some people would argue that dieters seem superficial and excessive, so we assume that they could tell us little about ourselves. It could also be argued that dieting is merely one aspect of people's lives, and that people are defined more accurately by occupation (firefighter, lumberjack, miner) or ethnicity (Anglo, African, Native American) rather than by body type. I disagree. We are our bodies. As one dieter puts it, "That crap that when you are fat you are still you—bullshit! My friends would not know how to handle it. People relate to you differently. Your body, your physical self, shapes your life experiences."[3]

I collected twenty-five written interviews from dieters who did not wish to be taped and fifty-five tape-recorded interviews, and I received twenty completed questionnaires from absent dieters who had once been on the Rice Diet. All names, occupations, and hometowns, except for those of the medical staff, have been changed.

The purpose of collecting these stories is to frame the experiences and expectations of diet culture. Telling and retelling these diet testimonies maintains the power and tradition of the Rice Diet. Since the testimonies are public statements of personal involvement, they evolve over time to fit a type of Ricer narrative role model. There is a relationship between the belief system Ricers reveal in their personal stories and the group's rules for testimony. Ricer narratives are a response to the structural conditions of this belief system.

I interviewed many more women than men because the ratio of women to men on diet programs in Durham is four to one. This reflects the gender ratio of the national population of dieters. Female dieters were easier to interview. Often, they heard of me through word of mouth and were very open to the interview process. They did not hesitate to reveal their personal struggles with weight. Women were anxious to tell someone about their involvement with diet culture. They were knowledgeable about the health risks that obesity poses to women and were aware that thirty-five to fifty percent of the adult female population is considered moderately to morbidly obese. Still, every woman's primary concern was with physical appearance rather than health. They wanted to be thin to look acceptable. Health was a secondary consideration.

Women were thrilled to be in Durham and have the opportunity to focus all their attention on dieting. They loved Durham and made lifelong friends while on the Rice Diet. They viewed Durham as one big sorority house. The women I interviewed saw dieting as a social event. They ate, exercised, and walked together every day. Yet all the women I interviewed felt guilty for leaving families and friends behind at home. Many were worried about the money and time they were spending on the Rice Diet and felt that they didn't have the right to be in Durham. Most felt guilty and even silly for putting their own needs before those of their husbands and children.

Every woman's family asked the same questions: Why couldn't she lose weight at home? It would be so much cheaper and easier for the family. Why did she have to travel to Durham, North Carolina, to eat rice and fruit? Couldn't she do that at home? There are Weight Watchers meetings everywhere and the majority of participants are women. Couldn't she find the support and camaraderie she needed at Weight Watchers? A reasonable, well-adjusted person could. A person who just put her mind to it could lose weight anywhere. What was the magic of Durham?

Every woman interviewed brought a burden of mixed feelings to the Rice Diet. All were successful in their careers, yet they didn't seem concerned about how their careers might suffer during their extended stays in Durham. They spoke of their anxieties about leaving loved ones, worried about how their families would cope without them.

Although the women I spoke with defined themselves by their relationships and connections rather than by their careers, the men I interviewed had the opposite priority. They spoke first of their fear of leaving jobs or businesses unattended, and later mentioned concern for their families. Men defined themselves by their professions. Their family and friends, though important, were secondary to career and business needs. The men's families had urged them to come to Durham to diet. The men themselves were reluctant and resented others for suggesting it. Only when they ran out of options did they find their way to the Rice Diet.

Men are rarer in diet culture and more difficult to interview. I had to find them; they didn't come to me. When I could get a man to agree to an interview, he would usually dictate the terms. He would pick the time and site of the interview and would select which of my questions he would answer. Only after several follow-up meetings would he relax enough to allow me to direct the interview.

Even though every man I interviewed was or had been obese, all of them were initially reluctant to admit that they had a weight problem. The dominant emotion I encountered when interviewing men was anger. Men were mad about being fat and loathed the notion that they had to diet to lose weight. They felt that obesity was a curse that had descended upon them. They raged at the injustice of it.

Everyone I interviewed, male or female, felt that the Rice Diet was ground zero for dieters. Weight loss was a war with a beginning and an end. The final battle was the Rice Diet, where one triumphed over obesity or was killed by it. I too felt that way when I began the Rice Diet. I still consider myself a Ricer. If only in my mind, I still try to adhere to the principles of the Diet.

The Dieters I interviewed ranged in age from seventeen to eighty-five. Some were first-time Ricers, brand new to Durham, while others were repeater Ricers and owned homes near the Rice House. One informant was a fifth-generation Ricer. All of them saw themselves as part of a greater diet culture that existed parallel to the mainstream thin culture. All saw Durham as the physical and symbolic capital of the ultimate dieting adventure. Their words speak of the breadth of the dieting experience and the formation of a thriving community of fellow dieters. The following chapters will take you on a journey deep into diet culture.

one Fat Like Me

I've always been a big girl. So I've led a different kind of life than normal-weight or thin girls do. Almost from birth, I knew that my body was wrong and even threatening to others. What is personal and private to most people—the body—was in my case open to unsolicited comments, helpful advice, painful ridicule, and sometimes violence from the general public.

Roly Poly, Daddy's little fatty—that was me. I was a plump baby for 1953: eight pounds, twelve ounces. My father was thin when I was young, and loved to rock his Roly Poly and coo lullabies to me. To him, you were either fat or thin and there was nothing anyone could do about it one way or another. But he wasn't fat, so he had no idea what life had in store for his chubby daughter.

My mother, however, had often been overweight in adulthood and was well aware of the consequences of obesity and the type of life that lay ahead of me. She dragged me from one fat doctor to another in the hope that there was a medical cure for my excessive and unruly flesh. My first memory of a doctor is the one who warned me not to eat any fatty meat, dairy products, or anything white: sugar, flour, or bread. He told me that if I didn't do this, I would grow up to be fat and no one would like me. I received my first prescription for diet pills—amphetamines—when I was eight years old, along with the classic food exchange diet sheet, and the admonition to go and eat no more.

This was in the early 1960s, and experts in the burgeoning field of childhood obesity believed that excess weight was the result of too many calories and too little exercise. It was a symbol of a weakening America. President John F. Kennedy had challenged a nation on its apparent laziness and poor physical conditioning, and public health advocates responded by prescribing a curriculum of calisthenics and strength tests, along with weight charts, for all public schools. Fat camps sprang up around the nation to shape up the country's overweight youth, and slick brochures from nearby camps, Weight Watchers notices, and Lane Bryant Chubbette advertisements soon jammed our mailbox. Once a month I would receive a Chubbette newsletter full of tips on how to appear slimmer, taller, and more confident—mostly by wearing black and vertical stripes and purchasing their advertised foundation garments. I was eight years old when I got my first training bra. My mother ordered it through the mail along with a panty girdle with slimming thigh panels. I remember the humiliation of putting them on and parading in front of my mother and our concerned next-door neighbor, Mrs. Levine. They both worried and fretted over my bulging body—I looked like a beach ball with legs. They discussed how I had no prospects for dating because I was so fat. They nodded their heads, agreeing that I would never amount to much. They ate donuts and coffee cake and drank Tab while I changed into and out of the outfits my mother had purchased for me.

Why couldn't I be like my older sister? She was thin. Tall, thin, blonde, and athletic. She dated the captain of the football team. All her friends and boyfriends looked as if they had stepped out of a Pepsi commercial. She was young and modern looking. She could wear shorts, halter tops, and tight-ribbed knit dresses. Her thighs never jiggled or rubbed together. Each fall before the beginning of school, we would go on a shopping trip to buy school clothes for the coming year. My sister got beautiful lingerie: ruffled pettipants, black lace slips, sheer bras, babydoll pajamas, and bikini underwear. I got A-line slips, industrial-strength cotton bras with circular stitching around the pointed cups, and big white brief-style underwear that came three to a package. My sister got miniskirts with matching sweaters and a pair of white go-go boots that zipped up the back. I got big black jumpers with white piping around the neck to draw attention upward to my face and away from my hips. We couldn't find any boots that would fit me because my calves were so large. I ended up trudging through the midwestern snows in my mother's old overshoes.

I learned from the Chubbette newsletters that the only way I would negotiate myself through the world was by camouflage and proper foundation garments. I would encase myself in nylon and Lycra each day for school: bra, girdle with garter clips, nylon stockings under my knee-highs because the stockings helped to hold in my jiggly flesh, taffeta full-length slip over all of that (the newsletters instructed that one must wear taffeta because it does not cling to the body, but merely skims it) and finally my dress—tentlike, in black, brown, or navy blue. The dress inevitably had a Peter Pan collar with a big floppy bow. I looked like some bizarre present. Every part of me that could be restrained, was. I could barely move, and there was always a part of my flesh that would not stay in place: A belly that would flop out over my many waistbands and rub against the elastic until a blood blister formed. Breast tissue that couldn't be contained by the training bra puffed out under my arms and irritated me most of the day, eventually creating a red, angry heat rash. The tops of my thighs seeped between my stockings and girdle, rubbing my skin raw by the end of the day. Even on the coolest days I was always hot and tired because I wore so many undergarments.

One edition of the newsletter told the story of a Miss America who was once a Chubbette too, but through hard work, perseverance, belief in God, and strict food monitoring grew up to become the crown princess of the United States. I got a free calorie book with that newsletter and an autographed picture of Miss America. I pinned her photo to my bulletin board, but I had no real hope that I would grow up to be a princess. I just knew I would never be thin. I was out of step with the rest of the world. America was getting lean and competitive.

I flunked the physical tests in school, scored in the dangerously overweight area of the weight chart, and tossed the food exchange lists the doctor gave me but kept the diet pills. I loved the way they made me feel: like I was zooming through space with my heart beating wildly in my ears. Yet the pills had no effect on my appetite, and my body remained fat.

I starved all through grade school, with my little diet sack lunch: one three-ounce apple without the peel, one-fourth cup of tuna fish without mayonnaise on one slice of plain Roman Meal bread, and a jumble of carrots and celery sticks. In the cafeteria, I bought a half-pint of skim milk and sat alone at a lunchroom table while all around me children gobbled down Fritos, peanut butter sandwiches, and Snickers bars. My teachers, all slim and young, sometimes sat with me and sipped their cans of Chocolate Malt Sego, Carnation Instant Slender, Tab, or Fresca and shared their dieting tips. They were nice to me and urged me to get thin at any cost.

On my tenth birthday, I had a slice of angel food cake and one-half cup of ice milk, while my guests had a bakery-made yellow cake with roses made from sugar frosting accompanied by French vanilla ice cream hand-packed from Baskin-Robbins. My life was one long denial of what I desired most—unlimited, calorie-laden, forbidden food. I became a secret eater.

By day, I was the perfect dieter and dutifully recorded in my Weight Watchers calorie ledger every morsel of food and ounce of liquid that passed through my hungry mouth. On paper my dieting was a success. At night, when the house was asleep, I pulled out my secret cache of food from behind my bookcase. The chips, salty and crisp in their cellophane bags, tasted bitter and sweet at the same time. The M&Ms, which always followed the chips, carried that sweetness even higher. I ate quickly and silently. I ate to the point where I would begin to relax inside, let go of the discipline of the dieting day, and allow the pleasure of the food to wash over me. It felt as if I were falling through an endless tunnel, and I enjoyed that feeling. I ate until my gnawing hunger was abated, and I felt good, whole, and complete until the next time. I remember slipping into the family room late at night and watching Jack

Paar interview an ex-fatty who went on the Rice Diet and lost a tremendous amount of weight. I was lying on the couch, sneaking handfuls of Kitty Klover potato chips from a bag I had hidden under a pillow, and thinking, one day that will be me. One day I too will go to Durham.

In fifth grade, our class was selected to put on a folk-dancing event for the whole school. We all had to wear costumes that our teacher selected for us. The girls were supposed to wear frilly white blouses, black short skirts, and lavender cummerbunds around their tiny waists, but my waist wasn't tiny. The costumes came and, of course, mine didn't fit. My mother had to take me to a seamstress and have a costume made for me. It looked like the other girls', but wasn't the same. I refused to wear it. In fact, I refused to be in the performance at all. I didn't want people laughing and pointing at the fat girl who was sweating to death in her white blouse, wool skirt, and elastic foundation garments. I didn't want to humiliate myself in front of the whole school. My mother came to school and met with my teacher. She asked that I be let off the hook and allowed to make up for it some other way.

My teacher told her that I must learn to accept the consequences of obesity if I was going to overeat. Simple as that. My overweight mother slumped home without protest. I had to dance in the event. They paired me up with Mark Overton, another fatty, and we looked like a pair of dancing bears as we glided across the auditorium floor. The audience laughed and clapped, and my teacher told me that I did a good job considering where I was coming from. My parents didn't attend the performance. They didn't want to hear people ridiculing their fat daughter. Mark later shared a Three Musketeers bar with me as we waited in the dark for our parents to pick us up.

Life was one long stretch of weight gain, dieting, weight loss, and even more weight gain accompanied by an overarching cloud of depression. I was tired all the time. I was either going on a new diet prescription or coming off one. I was running to an exercise class or collapsing on the couch exhausted from attending one. I tried to eat only when I was hungry, after I'd heard my stomach growl at least three times. Then I would eat just until I was sated. Sometimes I would chew the food, then spit it out. I would get motivated to go on a diet, force myself to do it, lose weight, and immediately rebound with even more weight gain. Fortunately, I had more success in other areas—school, music, church, friends—but my dream of a life of thinness and acceptance was out of reach. To the world, I was happy, cheerful, accommodating, pleasantly plump, even charming with a pretty face and a beautiful smile. Many fat girls are told they have these attributes, and we live in the hope that one day our bodies will transform and be aligned with our waiting faces. I always hated this compliment and felt as if my head had accidentally been placed on the wrong body. I knew that my body would never be pretty like my face, no matter how little I ate.

Parents and teachers and old people loved me. I was gracious and well-mannered. I cleaned the chalkboards after school and did errands for people. My friends liked me, and I took it as a personal mission to convince people to care about me and allow me to hang around with them even though they were disgusted by my size. I figured that if I made top grades, performed the best, and was the funniest, wittiest, and wildest, my weight would somehow fade away and the real me—the personality of me—would be enough for the world. I was the best friend, the class confidant, and the amateur therapist, with a sense of authority that most children didn't possess.

Sometimes, despite all my efforts, I found that some people just did not accept me. The summer before sixth grade, my parents took the family on a train trip to California. My parents' friends came to see us off at the station. My sister and I each had a little box lunch to take on the train. One of my father's co-workers pointed to mine and said, "You'll have that gone before the train pulls out of the station." Everybody laughed. My cheeks burned and I stared down at my shoes. He was right, too: as soon as I was on the train, I opened the box and finished the lunch just as the train whistle blew.

I would spend each summer with my grandparents in rural Missouri. I loved to go there because their house was a sanctuary. There was no mention of dieting. I am convinced my grandparents had never even heard of it. Food was abundant and unrestricted. My step-grandfather would make me pancakes and French toast for breakfast. Dinner was the noon meal, the biggest meal of the day. We'd eat fried chicken or country-fried steak or catfish, mashed potatoes and gravy, tons of vegetables swimming in grease, hot biscuits with hand-churned butter and wild honey, sweetened ice tea by the mugful, and homemade peach cobbler with a crust made from rendered pork lard. My grandmother made cakes and cookies and homemade fudge and popcorn. All the neighborhood kids would come by and eat. My cousins, also chubbos, loved to visit my grandparents. They too were on Weight Watchers diets at home. They enjoyed the freedom to eat whatever they wanted without reprimand. My grandparents, great-aunts, great-uncles, and all their friends didn't consider weight an issue. They simply delighted in me. Perversely, I never gained weight in the summer despite all that food. Once home, I would return to my dieting regimen.

In sixth grade, a new girl was assigned the desk next to mine. She was tall and skinny—all legs. Her hair and skin were the beige-blonde of a Barbie doll. She took one look at me and announced in a loud voice, "You're fat!" All my classmates and my favorite teacher were watching me. I knew I could succumb to her criticism and lose my standing with my friends, or I could fight back. I took the heaviest book out of my desk—my science book—and smacked her across the forehead with it. The new girl went flying backward out of her chair and cracked her head on the cement floor. Not only was I fat, I was strong! I was suspended for a week. Nobody in my sixth-grade class called me fat again.

When I turned thirteen a miraculous thing happened. My lumpy, husky body gave way to curves and definition. I grew to five foot six, and my Lane Bryant Chubbette clothes hung on me like the tents they were. I had breasts, hips, a waist, and even hipbones emerging from my sea of flesh. I was still large for my age—a size nine—but I was shaped better. Men, not boys, immediately noticed, and my girlfriends' fathers would insist on driving me home at night and commenting to me in the car on my blooming and developing body. I was embarrassed and thrilled by their remarks and felt a growing potential of future power. That power lay in the shape of my body, as I had always known it would. I dieted furiously, and the weight slid off. In six months I was a size seven and strangers would stop their cars as I walked by just to tell me how my body pleased them.

For the first time in my life I had it all, including an appropriately sized body. I saw a future of unlimited possibilities. I believed I could do anything because I was thin and the momentum of the world was with me. Boys who had hurled spitballs at me and called me "fat ass" now wanted to date me and would wait around the bus stop until I appeared. I would find love letters from secret admirers stuffed in my desk drawers. Girls who wouldn't be caught dead with me the year before now wanted me to join their groups and attend their parties. I was picked to go out for cheerleading and the pep squad. I twirled a baton in a sequined bathing suit. I rode on the handlebars of bicycles as boys who pursued me pedaled by their friends' houses. I was pretty, popular, and getting thin. I had it made.

I even began to exercise in public. My parents joined the community pool and every summer afternoon I swam for hours until my arms and legs ached. I loved to swim. It was the only time I felt small. The water buoyed me up, and I could float and dream of what it was like to weigh so little. One day as I pulled myself out of the pool, one of the older popular boys called me over. He was surrounded by a bunch of good-looking, thin high school girls who wore tiny bikinis and had perfect tans. I was trembling as I walked up to the group. He pointed to me and said, "Kid, you have great legs, you'll grow up to be a looker." I was so flabbergasted I couldn't speak. I just stood there as he nodded appraisingly, and the girls looked anxious.

I ran home, locked the door to my room, and just sat there, stunned that somebody could find me so attractive. I was leaving my fat cocoon behind. I was thrilled and scared. What did it mean to be thin and desired? Would I fall in love, get married to Prince Charming, and live happily ever after? And what would that mean? All I knew was that a young girl's key to happiness in the America of the 1960s was having a thin body.

When I was fourteen, my run of good luck ended. On the first date I was allowed to have, I was kidnapped, raped, and abandoned one hundred miles from my home. The police officers who interviewed me told me that the reason I was raped was that I was asking for it. "Just look at you," they said. "Look at that body and how you show it off. What kind of girl wears white shorts and a tank top? What kind of girl wears colored underwear? You got what you deserved." This was 1968, before shield laws were introduced to protect victims of rape. The policeman leaned over and asked me if I had experienced orgasm when I was raped. I had no idea what he was talking about. I went home and looked it up in the dictionary. The definition read "experience of extreme pleasure." I didn't experience any pleasure—just horror.

The state's attorney told me that when it was my time to go on the witness stand I had to be pure in mind, body, and spirit. I could wear no makeup, and had to pull my long hair back from my shoulders. I was instructed to wear a long plain skirt with flat shoes and a simple blouse. I was to do nothing that would emphasize my figure. My body, my looks, would decide the case. We never went to trial. I barely made it through the preliminary hearing, where I was positioned not five feet away from the man who had raped me. I cried through the entire hearing, and the charges against him were dismissed.

I gained seventy pounds within the two months following the rape. I never again felt the freedom, power, and pride in my body—and the belief in my unlimited abilities—that I had when I was fourteen, thin, and a virgin. The weight took me out of the dating pool, and men left me alone. I didn't want anyone's attention. I was afraid of it.

In high school, I went back to the role of good friend and confidant to the world. My desire for good grades, church activities, and the pursuit of music ended—but not my quest for thinness. Luckily, it was the late '60s and early '70s, and although there were no real places for fat girls in the dominant culture of mainstream white America, I found a niche in the counterculture. I was hippie momma, earth mother, big sister, and cushy tushy. I made love and not war—a lot. Boys seemed to think I was some kind of fertility doll, and because I was fat they thought I was an easy lay. Dopers would always ask me to score some speed for them, black beauties and yellow jackets. They assumed that since I was fat, I could get diet pills from doctors, and usually I could. I wouldn't even have to ask for the prescription. A doctor would take one look and hand me a prescription with an unlimited amount of refills. I wore long flowing dresses that covered my big body, but this time without the elastic foundation garments. My breasts were braless. For the first time, I felt comfortable in my clothes. Nothing itched, or clung, or chafed.

I still couldn't stand to have attention directed toward me. In my high school drama class we were each required to put on a one-act play. When it came my time to perform, I couldn't do it. I conveniently got sick. My mother again went to school and asked my teacher to let me out of the required performance. This time my teacher was understanding. She said I should try it, but if I didn't think I could do it, I didn't have to. I practiced each evening in front of a mirror. I thought I would use my vulnerability instead of hiding it. I performed Edward Albee's *The Sand Box* and got a standing ovation. I loved the applause, but I knew that I didn't deserve it because I was fat.

I still ate nothing in public, nor during the day. I also found a friend in weight loss—drugs. Unlike the amphetamines of my grade school years, drugs in high school worked, especially cocaine. With coke, the gnawing hunger for food left me, and I could go days without eating anything. I did lose weight and people commented on my willpower, strength, and hollow cheekbones. I was actually thin for a while and could squeeze into size nine jeans—even size seven, if a friend sat on one of my hipbones and squished me together as I tugged the zipper up one inch and one breath at a time. All the girls I knew, fat or thin, did drugs for their weight-loss effects. We were a generation dedicated to the ideal woman of the early 1970s. We were strong, invincible women who could, thanks to the women's movement, be anything we wanted to be. What we wanted most of all was to be thin. As our selection of career and educational opportunities widened, our physical ideals narrowed. There were no fat, successful role models. Farrah Fawcett's body—posters of which covered teenage boys' bedroom walls—was rail thin. Even Gloria Steinem, the icon of the women's movement, was lean. There were no fat poster girls, no plump leaders.

Eventually, the power of coke was eroded by the superior strength of my hunger and my uncooperative metabolism. I began to gain weight. I knew my chemically induced run of weight loss was over. By my senior year of college I accepted the fact that I was permanently fat and would grow even more so until one day my heart would supernova in a massive coronary. I weighed almost one hundred pounds more than my ideal body weight.

I became a very good actress. I learned to negotiate my immense flesh through a daily gauntlet of environmental and social obstacles. I pretended to be happy and even content with my existence. I wouldn't let mere weight stop me from having a good time. I went to the beach and proudly strolled the boardwalk in defiance of the thin passersby. I was dying inside, but nevertheless I forced myself to do it. I graduated from college, worked for a while, then moved across the country and gained even more weight.

I went to doctors constantly. I kept trying to find a reason for my weight, trying to figure out why I couldn't stick to a diet, couldn't keep the weight off, and couldn't stop thinking about food. I knew that there had to be some reason for it, some biochemical lever that was stuck in the wrong position. Most doctors were repulsed by me, loathed the fat, and looked upon me with a mixture of pity and revulsion. I kept going to them and kept following the twelve-hundred-calorie exchange diet they received from the American Dietetic Association—the same diet I'd endured when I was eight years old. I did all the right things and just got fatter.

Oh, I tried all the diets—the new ones, the old standbys, the popular magazine diets, the doctor-certified diets, the hospital-based fasts—tried them all. I followed Oprah on her Optifast, and watched her reach her goal weight on national television. I never reached mine. I made the right sounds and motions and forked over my hard-earned money from my lousy job to buy yet another useless and boring diet book, or sign up for yet another diet program administered by some perky, tiny ex-cheerleader who made a living telling fat girls that we just had to try harder, apply ourselves, and of course, purchase her tasty prepackaged and calorie-restricted dinners, so we too could be on the beach in a bikini by next summer.

As my body expanded, my environment grew smaller. The world was a threatening arena of too-tight spaces and too-small chairs. Worse than the physical pain and public embarrassment of my obesity was the constant awareness that I was always settling for much less than what I truly wanted in life. I knew there was no way I could—with my enormous body—get a good job, a good opportunity, or a good relationship. Fat people suffer discrimination in all areas of life. Fat women, especially, feel the brunt of such discrimination. They make less money, marry less often or not at all, and are more likely to be denied admission into colleges than thinner women with similar backgrounds. We are a nation that defines ability by physical shape.

We are obsessed with weight. It still remains that "the world loves you thin, and hates you fat,"[4] as writer and dieter Judy Moscovitz pointed out to me. Yet we are also a nation of fat people and getting fatter with each passing year. In 1994, the *Journal of the American Medical Association* reported that there had been a substantial increase in the number of overweight adults since 1960.[5] In 2001, it is estimated that over half of all U.S. citizens aged twenty and over are medically overweight (up to thirty pounds over ideal body weight). The number of obese Americans (thirty pounds or more over ideal body weight) rose from twelve percent in 1991 to nearly eighteen percent in 1998. Sixty-three percent of all American men and fifty-five percent of women over the age of twenty-five are obese or overweight—the highest rate ever recorded. The fastest increase in national weight gain has occurred within the last five years. So has an increase in spending in the diet industry. We are a people who exercise more, eat less fat, and gain more weight at a faster rate than any other in recorded history. Historian and writer Roberta Pollack Seid, in her book *Never Too Thin: Why Women Are at War With Their Bodies,* asserts that America's creed is, "I watch my weight, eat right, and exercise."[6] Yet this idea sends out conflicting messages; our creed has spawned a series of paradoxes. We live in a country that supposedly celebrates diversity, but we have a very narrow range of acceptable body types. We live in a nation of plentiful food, but we are urged not to partake of much of it. We are liberated women who are enslaved by the bathroom scale.

I was living the paradoxes. By the time I was thirty years old I had done everything I could think of to lose weight. When I couldn't lower my weight, I struggled to raise my self-esteem, and I read book after book on how to love myself and accept my body no matter how large it was. I read magazines such as *Radiance*, *Mode*, and *Big, Beautiful Woman*, and I forced myself to go to eating and self-esteem workshops. Nothing worked, and it didn't matter anymore. I didn't care about anything at all—not work, not my family or my friends. Living day to day was like sleepwalking: the days passed, but I had no recollection of them. I still feebly attempted to follow a diet program or two. I sought out psychiatrists and physiologists on occasion, searched medical literature for guidance and advice, and took courses in nutrition even though a lifetime of dieting had given me a working knowledge of the calorie, sodium, and fat content of anything edible, but I had no zest for anything. I knew, really knew in my viscera, that my life was coming to an end, and I was slowly but perceptibly leaving this world behind. I knew I was dying. As I sat on my patio that one night so long ago, screaming one last plea to the powers that be in this universe, I knew I would die or go to Durham. Just like that, I knew that in Durham, North Carolina, I would find one last chance for a new, authentic, thin life.

I had thought about going to Durham many times in my life. I would write long sorrowful letters to the Duke University Medical Center and the Rice Diet program about my massive weight and my useless attempts to control it. Looking back, those letters were my first steps to Durham. Duke would, in response, send form letters instructing me to call for an appointment and send them my health insurance information as quickly as possible. Duke also warned me about the cost in time, money, and commitment. Their philosophy was that obesity is a multidimensional disease and must be approached in a scientific manner, without the interruptions of work or family.

Dr. Kempner, the founder of the Rice Diet, emphasized this in his letter to prospective dieters: "We know this treatment is time-consuming and an inconvenient nuisance, but it should be done in a scientific way and not in a hit-or-miss fashion according to the patient's own taste and preference. In spite of everything, it is the lesser evil."[7] I would think about going and then put the Duke letter away in a file. The money involved was overwhelming to me—approximately $300 a week at that time, plus living and transportation expenses. Where would I get that kind of money? How could I just move clear across the country for something as elusive to me as weight loss?

I told my family about Durham, and they assured me that I could lose weight in California as well as I could in North Carolina. They told me all I had to do was try harder, apply myself. Use some self-discipline. They were not going to give me any money to go to Durham to diet. They thought it was a silly idea. Obviously, they were out of touch with reality. They had been witnesses to my dieting failures for my entire life, yet were somehow convinced that I could lose weight at home if I just tried one more time.

My father told me to just get over it. Accept the fact that I was fat, and accept my role in life. My brother was in the military and assumed that I should apply more discipline to my eating behaviors. My sister was thin and away from home, living her own life, and my mother was in denial about the impact of weight. She told me I should focus on my inner beauty rather than change my outer appearance. I even tried to discuss the idea with my family doctor. He laughed in my face. Told me that it was preposterous and even silly. He knew I couldn't do it—knew I could not lose weight. This treatment was nothing new to me. Most of the doctors I have encountered throughout my life felt the same way.

I wanted to go to Durham, but I had too much to attend to first. I had a job—albeit a low-paying one that I didn't like but didn't actually hate—and a mediocre job was better than having no job. Besides, who would hire me at my weight? I should have been grateful for any job—didn't study after study tell us that employers hate to hire fat people, especially women? I should have been thankful that anyone would give a job to someone as overweight as I was.

My whole life was conditioned to accept less and not cause a stir. Be quiet, be content, accept yourself. Don't draw attention—hard to do when you are the biggest object in a room.

I had a relationship that I valued, although it was lousier than my job—but hey, I was fat and he was okay, not that bad, and who else would go out with a fat girl? I had family and friends. My family used me as a buffer for their own emotional problems, a night-duty nurse, and a housekeeper, and my friends saw me as the fat and faithful guest who would come early to set up for a party and stay late to clean up. I was the friend who would always remember birthdays, anniversaries, and other people's celebrations. Why not? I didn't have anything of my own to celebrate, and I saw it as some sort of duty to stand at the ready to serve in other people's lives.

I had an existence, damn it—an awful one, but a busy one—and I didn't have the time or money to go to Durham and eat rice and fruit for a year or more on some expensive diet program. Besides, I knew deep down that I truly didn't deserve the opportunity that Durham represented. I didn't deserve happiness or freedom. I didn't deserve to be thin because I believed I was a bad, useless, and worthless human being who was living a God-given perfectly pointless existence. I felt that I was being punished for some deep, unforgivable, and unknowable sin, and that's why I was cursed with a faulty, uncooperative metabolism and layers of resulting fat. God hated me and, like, everyone else, was repulsed by my body.

I also believed that there was no way I could actually lose the weight. No way. All my diet experience had taught me this. My friends, my family, and those smug doctors believed it, too. I knew I could never lose weight, and if I did, the loss would be temporary at best. Still, some part of me had hope that Durham actually was the land of miracles.

I made the call to Duke Medical Center, and two weeks later was sitting in the dining room of the dilapidated old Rice House, eating rice and fruit and feeling like it was the most satisfying meal I'd ever had.

two

Diet Capital of the World

I had known about Durham most of my life. I saw newly thin people interviewed on late-night talk shows about their tremendous and speedy weight loss at the Rice House. I read in my mother's *Good Housekeeping* magazine about important people who lost weight in Durham. I was about eight years old at the time, but the article made an impression on me. I knew celebrities, the rich and famous, and the extremely wealthy went to Durham to lose weight, but I didn't think average fat people like me went there. How could we? Who but the wealthy could afford the Rice Diet? How could poor and middle-class people find the time and money to go to Durham? To me, Durham remained a dream, a distant hope of someday. When my ship came in and I got rich, I would go to the Rice House, lose all my weight, and never get fat again. I would be cured—if only I could find the time and money.

I knew it would not happen. I never heard of people like me going to Durham. Then I read *The Rice Diet Report* by Judy Moscovitz. Judy detailed her phenomenal weight loss on the Rice Diet and her sacrifice to get there. She sold all her furniture, books, and records—everything she owned—to finance her stay in Durham. She quit her profession and left her family. She was not rich or famous or even sure she would make it at the Rice House, but she went anyway. Her book did not show a picture of her before the

Rice Diet, but her thin photograph on the back cover was enough to convince me. If someone like Judy could sell everything for the chance to lose weight in Durham, so could I. It could happen to me.

After I had the epiphany on the patio of my house about my life and the devastating role fat played in it, I wrote to the Rice Diet requesting that I be admitted as a patient. They, in turn, sent me a colorful brochure hailing the preeminence of Duke University Medical Center and extolling the charms of Durham. I contacted the Chamber of Commerce, and they sent me more brochures, a map, and a booklet of hotels, restaurants, and upcoming events in the area. The map depicted Durham as the center of the universe and Duke University as Durham's nucleus. The brochures pictured happy, healthy, slim people riding bicycles around Duke in the warm southern sun. The booklet was jammed with listings of interesting-sounding cultural happenings, nice hotels, and world-class restaurants. I looked at the glossy photos of people dining in those restaurants, really thin people eating beautifully arranged food. I would be like those people. I would get thin and ride a bicycle to many cultural events, and then go eat lovely food in starred restaurants. I would eat and never get fat, because once I did a tour of the Rice Diet, I would be thin forever. I would not regain any lost weight. I would remain thin because the Rice Diet would remove the curse of obesity. It would cleanse my chubby soul, and I would be born anew. I would be just like those slim celebrities on television who raved about their successful and permanent weight loss in Durham.

As I was driving east from California, the image of the mythical Durham kept coming to mind. After reading all those information packets sent to me by the Chamber of Commerce and Duke University, I was expecting Durham to be the land of enchantment. I thought it would shimmer with possibilities and actually rise up against the horizon like a beacon. In the brochures, Durham sounded like a genteel mid-sized city full of southern hospitality combined with the technology and brain power of Duke University. I thought Durham would be a lovely blend of the Old South (without slavery) and new, high-tech medicine. I believed that Durham would shine as the Emerald City in the Wizard of Oz, and I, like Dorothy, would find what I needed there. What I found when I turned off the I-40 ramp into the city of Durham was a dump.

I pulled into the parking lot of the Hampton Inn because their sign read "special rate for Ricers." That would be me. Soon I would be a Ricer. I arrived in August. The heat and humidity were so intense that the asphalt on the highway waffled in places. The air was so heavy it shimmered. I could not believe how hot it was. The brochure from the Chamber of Commerce had informed me that the average temperature was a comfortable 59.9 degrees. The bank sign across from the Hampton Inn showed a temperature reading of ninety-seven degrees. How could anybody, especially anybody fat, stand this kind of climate? I didn't see one person on the street, and no one was riding around on a bicycle. Durham looked like a ghost town.

Across from the motel was a strip mall with a pizza parlor, a yogurt shop, a Mexican café, a Greek restaurant, and a Shoney's with a day-long, all-you-can-eat breakfast bar. A half-mile past the mall was a street lined with every fast-food place imaginable: Dunkin' Donuts, KFC, Taco Bell, Pizza Hut, Wendy's, McDonald's, Chick-fil-A, Miami Subs, and more. A half-mile from the Rice House were even more fast food and chain restaurants: Golden Corral, Sizzler's Steak House, Captain D's, Pizza Hut, Pizza Villa, and Pizza Inn. These areas were known to dieters as Sin City and were constant reminders of cheap, forbidden, and anonymous food that was off-limits.

I found Durham to be a city of opposites. On one hand, it is the diet capital of the world. On the other hand, it has more cheap, fast, and available food than any place I have ever been. Food is everywhere in Durham and a constant source of forbidden pleasure and pain. Food courts at the malls hire workers who plead with shoppers to sample their free eats. Upscale grocery stores have in-house displays of everything from gourmet chocolates to cheese trays—all for the taking. Churches welcome dieters of all faiths with ham biscuits and cheese-grits casseroles for breakfast. I discovered the abundance of food the day I arrived. I got in early and drove around to try to get oriented. I went to the mall to kill time and to be around people. I knew no one in Durham. I declined all offers of food. Curiously,

I had no hunger. Perhaps the power of the diet capital of the world was already working its magic.

The Durham I encountered was not at all as I had pictured in my mind, nor was it anything like those glossy brochures. It was not Old South meets high tech, but uneven and organic. Durham seemed to have no plan to it, no structure, but it did have a rhythm. I would find that out later.

Coming from Sacramento, I was used to flat, dry towns that lay on a square, with each street framing the initial square. Durham was nothing like that. It seemed to ramble on like a weedy plant. Streets changed their names without reason and meandered off into nowhere. Many roads were unpaved. Nothing seemed well thought out. Everything looked random and incomplete. Old mansions from a forgotten era, now chopped into rentals, stood side by side with little bungalows. Good sections were backed up to bad ones. There seemed to be no zoning regulations. Duke University, with its imitation Oxford setting, was plunked down in a field of parking lots. Duke appeared to be the center of Durham and was ringed by old neighborhoods and hollyhocks. Radiating out from Duke were strip malls and suburbs. Farther out still were abandoned tobacco barns and empty farmhouses, reminders of Durham's agrarian past.

Durham was a shock to my dry, brown, western sensibilities. The city was so green, it was as if I had taken some hallucinogen to enhance my senses. It vibrated green color everywhere. Maybe it truly was the Emerald City. Green overlapping trees draped the broken sidewalks. Houses were hidden by a guard of leaves. Abandoned buildings and forgotten cars were shot through with green kudzu. Green weeds poked through crumbling walls. Something green was growing all over the city. It was almost primitive in its fecundity. Everything was alive.

The smell of all that greenery was that of rotting vegetation and mold that lingered even in the dead of winter. Added to it was the scent of honeysuckle in the early spring, almost sickening in its sweetness. Layered on all of these smells was the faint, sweet, clean whiff of curing tobacco.

On my third morning in Durham, I went to the Rice Diet Clinic for my preliminary tests. Two other initiates joined me. One was from

Florida and the other from New York. We were all thrilled to be going on the Rice Diet and pledged to each other that we would get thin and stay that way. After going through a battery of screening exams, including a blood oxygen test and a "before" photo session, I was told to show up at the Rice House for meals. That was it. There was no information packet, no wad of material like I used to get at Weight Watchers. The nurse told me to go eat at the Rice House and not leave until I weighed 112 pounds—Duke's goal weight for me. Since I was five foot six, I knew I would never weigh so little and would be in Durham eating rice and fruit forever.

Before I started the Diet, I moved out of the Hampton Inn into my car. I was prepared to sleep in it if necessary. To stay in a motel for any length of time, even with Ricer rates, was too costly. Luckily, I found an inexpensive place to live immediately. From the Rice Diet Clinic, I got a list of widows willing to rent out rooms to Ricers. I located one who lived in a house on the corner of Trinity and Mangum streets: two miles from the Wall, two blocks from the Rice House, and at the crest of Cardiac Hill. The Wall is the stone fence that surrounds Duke's east campus. Ricers walk around this wall for exercise. New Ricers especially can be seen at the Wall. Returning Ricers who have gained weight and lost touch with diet culture walk the wall to remind themselves of who they are. Cardiac Hill is the long, steep climb up Trinity Avenue from Duke Street. This is the last trek before the Rice House.

I learned all of these terms from my landlady, Mrs. Ethylene Cole. She had been renting to Ricers for over forty years and knew everything there was to know about diets, dieters, and the doctors of Duke. Although she'd only left the state once in her life, she received a worldwide education from her renters. She told me that she expected the best behavior from her renters and would not allow any overnight male guests. I assured her I would not have any. She sighed and said, "They all do. After fifty pounds you'll be dancing every night at the Crisco Disco in a leather miniskirt or hanging out at the bar at the Sheraton."[8] That was my first inkling that there was more to Durham than I had thought.

The first time I saw the Rice House I was shocked. I knew it would not be a spa or a resort, but I didn't know it would be as run down as it was. (When I started at the Rice House, it was located at 1111 Mangum Street. At times it has had other locations. Currently it is on Cole Mill Road.) The Rice House itself was a large old building that had seen better days. The big wraparound porch was sagging in places from years of pounding by the obese. The chairs on the porch were rusted, warped with age and abuse, and full of Ricers.

I remember thinking that I had made some kind of mistake. I was fat, yes, but these people were huge. Maybe I should have tried Weight Watchers one more time. Perhaps I was in the wrong place. Jumbos and Jumboettes were jammed into rickety gliders and sofas. Flesh was abundant, hanging off of seats and squishing out of the backs of chairs. Everyone wore shorts. In my entire life, I had never seen so many fat people in shorts, and they were not a bit concerned about it. I felt like I had walked onto the set of some strange movie. I didn't know that many fat people existed! It was like looking in a mirror. I was frightened and disturbed, but at the same time I was relieved. I could let go and breathe. I was no longer the lone fat person. At the Rice House, fat was as common as dirt. I was just like everybody else. For the first time since I was raped, my body was normal.

I opened the old door of the Rice House and stepped into a parlor filled with old couches and cots and two sets of scales: one for people under three hundred pounds and one for those who were over. After I weighed in and a nurse took my blood pressure, I went to the dining room for breakfast. The dining room was just as dilapidated as the rest of the house. The tables were worn and the chairs precariously wobbly. The placemats, plates, and cups were paper. I sat down at one of the tables and a waitress brought me a tiny bowl of watery oatmeal and one half of a grapefruit. That was it. That was breakfast. I could not believe that this was the world-famous Rice Diet. Yet as I sat at that table and began talking to Ricers, I discovered the power of the simplicity—and even starkness—of the Diet and its surroundings. I heard stories of super dieters, the pathos of weight gain, the joys of redemption and goal weight, and the pitfalls of backsliding. I listened to the history of the Rice Diet and Durham's rise to diet capital of the world status. I began to learn about diet culture.

Four world-class diet programs have been established in Durham. The Rice Diet is the oldest, followed by the Duke Diet and Fitness Center (DFC), Structure House, and the Center for Living (CFL). All the diet programs except the Rice Diet began in the 1970s, and all four came out of programs at Duke University Medical Center. DFC, Structure House, and CFL have similar multidisciplinary approaches to dieting and oppose many of the Rice Diet precepts. Each, however, has a particular focus specific to its program for weight control. Structure House is the only one of the four major diet programs not owned by Duke University.

In 1939, Dr. Kempner originated the basic Rice Diet, which consisted of nothing but fruit, rice, and sugar. He treated his patients suffering from heart disease, kidney disease, and high blood pressure with a short course of the Diet. In 1942, a major breakthrough occurred by accident. According to the founding legend of the Rice Diet, which has been recounted by Ricers and doctors and in publications since the 1940s, Dr. Kempner instructed one of his patients to eat rice and fruit for two weeks and return to him for follow-up treatment. The patient, a North Carolina farmer's widow, did not understand Dr. Kempner's thick German accent and thought he had said two months instead of two weeks. At the end of two months, the widow returned with dramatic results. Her disease was gone, her heart size was normal, her blood pressure had stabilized, and, most importantly to the future of the Rice Diet, she had lost sixty pounds. This founding legend of diet culture is what brought us to Durham.

Dr. Walter J. Kempner was the founder and spiritual leader of diet culture. Without him there would have been no home for the obese, and no hope either. Many people also believe that without Dr. Kempner, Duke University Medical Center would have remained a minor regional hospital instead of becoming what it is today—a world center for medical research. Dr. Eugene A. Stead Jr., former chairman of the Department of Medicine at Duke, wrote that "Duke Hospital was just a small, regional medical center. It was the rise of Walter Kempner's Rice Diet program that really put Durham on the international map of medicine."[9]

I didn't meet the famous Dr. Kempner when I started his Rice Diet. He was still in Europe on his annual summer tour. Everyone was anxious for his return, and I looked forward to meeting him. As I heard more and more stories about him, I began to do research on Dr. Kempner and his deep and continuing influence on Duke. Kempner's lore could be found in the stories of his Ricers. I found the facts in Duke's archives.

Two fortuitous events helped hurl Duke to worldwide renown. The first was James B. Duke's founding of Duke University; Duke had enough money in 1924 to purchase the top academics of the world and bring them to Durham. The second was the rise of Nazi Germany. Scholars, doctors, and researchers anxious to leave Europe were financed by American philanthropic organizations. Dr. Kempner was among those brought over to America.

In 1934, Dr. Frederic Hanes, chairman of medicine at the newly established medical school at Duke, set out to make the Duke University School of Medicine a world-class medical center that specialized in research. His first step was to obtain a top-notch international faculty. He traveled the world searching for the most successful doctors involved in innovative research. While Dr. Hanes was trying to get the medical center off the ground, Dr. Kempner was at the Kaiser Wilhelm Institute for Cellular Physiology in Berlin, working with Dr. Otto Warburg, the 1931 Nobel laureate in biochemistry. As a medical student, Dr. Kempner's research was in cellular metabolism, oxygen tension, and renal physiology.

Kempner was born in Germany in 1903 and died in Durham in 1997. He is still listed in the Durham phone book. He was groomed for a life in medicine from the beginning. Each of his parents were doctors and trained as assistants to Robert Koch, discoverer of the tuberculosis bacillus, and each earned a national reputation for independent medical research. Kempner's father discovered a cure for botulism, and his mother made advances in the treatment of tuberculosis.

Kempner received his sense of discipline from his parents. He graduated first in his class and earned his medical degree in 1926. Around this time, he became a follower of the German poet Stefan George. George believed that a successful life could only be attained through discipline. Kempner became part of a group known as the George Kreis, or circle. In 1933, George fled Germany for

Switzerland, and Kempner followed. Years later in Durham, Kempner would develop his own circle of followers and prescribe discipline as the answer to all of life's problems—including obesity.

Dr. Kempner made a name for himself in Europe at a young age with his research in diabetes and kidney disease. Dr. Hanes heard about the research that Dr. Kempner was doing. He went to Germany and hired Kempner as the first salaried member of Duke's Department of Medicine. Kempner's responsibilities were teaching and medical research. He accepted the job on the conditions that he have free rein to conduct his research as he saw fit and that he be allowed three months off each summer to return to his beloved Europe. These unusual conditions attest to Dr. Kempner's many eccentricities and the power of his personality. A rumor from Ricer lore credits Dr. Hanes with smuggling money into Germany in the gas tank of a car so Kempner could escape before World War II broke out.

Wherever Dr. Kempner went, there was controversy. He was a member of the Duke Department of Medicine's teaching staff, yet he never taught a class or attended a faculty meeting. Dr. Stead remembers that "Dr. Kempner had made many enemies because he was honest and uncompromising and never spent a single hour of his life, except for some scientific talks on rare occasions, in any society or even in a committee meeting."[10] Why did Duke put up with such odd behavior? Because Kempner attracted worldwide attention with his research in kidney disease. Hiring Dr. Kempner was to transform the medical center from a regional hospital into an international one that attracted patients and practitioners from all over the globe. Those in power at Duke believed that Dr. Kempner would become a Nobel prize candidate. Instead, he became the king of diet culture.

Kempner did not set out to be a diet doctor. His interest was in the treatment of chronic disease. He was the first doctor—long before Nathan Pritikin and Dr. Dean Ornish—to use food as a therapeutic intervention and to study the results of the regulation of the type and quantity of food on the body's ability to heal itself. In 1939, he was the first doctor in America to prescribe the short-term use of a low-sodium, low-fat, low-protein diet, which came to be known as the Rice Diet. It was the first effective treatment for hypertension, kidney dysfunction, elevated cholesterol, and heart disease.

At that time, a diagnosis of hypertension was a death sentence. Ninety percent of hypertension patients died within two years of diagnosis. Most doctors believed there was no effective treatment or cure. Dr. Kempner thought otherwise and applied the Rice Diet with amazing results. His conclusions became the basis for modern therapy. In 1944, Kempner presented his clinical findings to the American Heart Association meeting in Chicago. The results were revolutionary. He documented rapid improvements in kidney dysfunction, hypertension, high cholesterol, and cardiovascular disease and proved that these chronic conditions could be stopped or even reversed. His research results were met with skepticism, anger, and controversy. His findings contradicted established medical theories. Also, Kempner refused to follow standard scientific procedure by using a control group to test his results. He argued was that it was unethical to deny patients the benefits of his discoveries by placing a portion of them in a control group. He felt that the well-being of his patients was more important than adherence to scientific research practices.

However, according to Duke University historian and Ricer James Gifford, Kempner's results were chiefly discounted because of the xenophobic attitudes of the American Heart Association. "Kempner was a person of German nationality working during and immediately after World War II. He was accused of falsifying his results."[11]

Dr. Kempner was not without his enemies, and his Teutonic manner, brilliant mind, and unusual habits were upsetting to many people. He never married; instead he surrounded himself with a dozen women, most of whom he brought over from Germany. He got them jobs in his labs, bought them houses and connected all the houses together through a series of walkways, took them on vacation, sent them to medical school, bought them cars and other gifts, and sometimes made them millionaires. He was often the object of suspicion and resentment.

A story from Ricer lore describes a time when Dr. Kempner

came to the attention of the local police. Every evening after dark, someone would knock once at Kempner's door and be quickly admitted. The blinds were drawn and no light could be seen from the street. No one would emerge until after midnight. Concerned that a German spy ring was being conducted under their very noses, the neighbors called the police and the FBI to ask them to investigate what was actually going on in Kempner's house. The stunned police learned that the German doctor and his associates gathered each night to play bridge, not to plot to overthrow the United States government.

In 1949, Dr. Kempner again presented his findings on the disappearance of congestive heart failure and the reversal of heart disease through the application of the Rice Diet. His results were rejected. By 1958, he had proven that the need for insulin in normalizing the blood sugar of a diabetic could be reduced or eliminated completely through strict adherence to the Rice Diet. Again, the medical community treated his findings with disdain. In response to Kempner's challenge, research groups at major teaching hospitals nationwide intensified their efforts to prove him wrong. However, their findings confirmed Kempner's research, and in 1991 the Physicians Committee for Responsible Medicine recommended a rice diet to reduce the risks of heart disease and cancer. Now everyone accepts as truth that diet and exercise are key elements in prevention and healing of major diseases.

Although the medical establishment downplayed Kempner's success, the media picked up the news, and soon very ill people began showing up in Durham asking for Dr. Kempner. According to Dr. Robert Rosati, Kempner's ideological twin and the current head of the Rice Diet, "Durham was just a podunk medical center in 1940, but people came here to get the Kempner treatment. He made this place internationally famous."[12] Very fat people also showed up in Durham. Obesity was and still is a very difficult condition to treat, and in the 1940s there was no established scientific approach to treatment until Dr. Kempner's Rice Diet emerged.

Dr. Kempner was the program's total and absolute head, and his influence is still powerfully felt in the Rice Diet community. His authority was supreme. As he told one potential Ricer, "If I ask you to eat wallpaper, you will eat wallpaper."[13] Kempner demanded compliance to the Diet and his directives. He dominated everyone around him.

Duke University Medical Center staff psychiatrist Kae Enright states that "the reason so many people came to Durham was Dr. Kempner. He represented the ultimate authority, the father figure who would reward us when we pleased him and punish us when we didn't."[14]

Sharon Ryan, a Ricer who came to the Rice Diet in the 1970s and stayed, sued Dr. Kempner and Duke University Medical Center for Kempner's alleged sexual misdeeds and mental domination. She claimed that while she was a Ricer she violated one of Dr. Kempner's rules by gaining weight. Under the guise of treatment, Kempner ordered Ms. Ryan to go into the examining room and expose her buttocks. Ms. Ryan did as she was told, and Dr. Kempner then whipped her with a riding crop. He immediately put his arms around her and embraced her. She became the lover, confidant, and virtual slave of Dr. Kempner for twenty-three years—so claimed Ms. Ryan.[15]

Kempner got her a job at the Rice House, and she entered his inner circle of the chosen few who surrounded him and reinforced his mystique. She lived in one of the many houses Kempner owned in Durham, dropped out of college, and spent all of her time following him around. Ryan claims that Kempner used an intense system of rewards and punishments, from gifts of cars, houses, and dream vacations to spankings. She believed Kempner to be Godlike and that without him she would die. Her license plate read "10/05/70"—the day she met Dr. Kempner.

Kempner flatly denied all charges. Duke did acknowledge that Dr. Kempner had used a riding crop on several patients in the past, but stopped it at the request of the university. Duke frames the use of physical punishment for weight loss as improper medical therapy, not sexual misconduct. Sharon Ryan insists that her relationship with Kempner was sexual and that sexual relations between them occurred frequently and everywhere. She says that they even had sex on Kempner's living room floor. Kempner's response was,

"I never had sex on the floor. My house has some nice couches and sofas. I would never have sex on the floor."[16]

The news of the lawsuit took the national papers by storm, and reporters, photographers, and television journalists appeared in Durham to interview anyone who had ever felt the sting of Dr. Kempner's infamous whip, or who would have liked to. The reaction of Rice Dieters, however, was lukewarm. While the world giggled about the carryings-on of fat people and their Herr Doktor in Durham, Ricers closed ranks.

The strength of the Rice Diet rested on the unique personality of Dr. Kempner. In theory, anyone could eat white rice and canned fruit at home and lose weight, but it was Kempner who ensured weight loss. He was relentlessly consistent in an ever-changing world, and there was something reassuring about that. He drove the same car, a black vintage Lincoln Continental with the top down, rain or shine. It was a gift from an adoring Ricer. He wore the same style of clothes every day. According to Ricer Al Goldstein, "The fat subculture is haunted by Dr. Kempner, a stern dictatorial man who always dressed the same way, in a blue blazer and white ducks—like someone's Nazi grandfather."[17]

Dr. Kempner would not have made it in the confessional world of today's America. He would not have been a good talk-show guest. He believed that introspection would not help a person lose weight, because knowing the problem and doing something about it are two completely different things. Dr. Kempner felt deeply that weight loss was the key to unlocking emotional problems. Change the body and the mind will follow: once the physical problems are gone, the emotional barriers will be easier to scale. Action precedes thought, not the other way around. To explain the ineffectiveness of psychotherapy, Dr. Kempner would tell Ricers this story: A man was on a twelfth-floor window ledge, ready to jump off. A Duke psychiatrist arrived and told the potential jumper to read chapter ten in his book on suicide prevention. The jumper didn't respond and moved closer to the edge. Finally, as a last resort, the psychiatrist called the Rice House. Dr. Kempner came at once, pushed the psychiatrist aside, pointed to the jumper and said, "Get off the ledge, you fool."[18]

Smart people, thought Dr. Kempner, were the worst dieters because they were constantly assessing the Diet rather than following it. He also believed that all dieters were liars and unable to be truthful about the amount of food they consumed, so he insisted on twice-weekly urine samples and daily weigh-ins. Being summoned by Dr. Kempner was like being sent to see the principal. The first thing out of his mouth to anyone, Ricer or not, was, "Did you lose [weight]?"

I spent the rest of August listening to Ricer stories and learning Ricer ways. By the time September came around and Dr. Kempner returned to the Rice House, I had lost almost twenty pounds. I was so tired of eating only rice and fruit. When I met Dr. Kempner he asked me, "Did you lose?" Yes, I said, and he took my hand. "Do it, do it, do it," he instructed me. Then he turned and walked away. That was my audience with the great man, and strangely it did its magic. I did what he said. I ate rice and fruit and when I couldn't look at rice anymore, I ate nothing at all. I continued to lose the weight. I believed I could. I believed I was called to Durham to do just that. After talking to other Ricers, I learned that we all thought that and felt deeply that we were called to dieting. Just like some people receive the call to a religious conversion or a vocation, or are prompted to go on a quest, dieters get the call to come to Durham.

three

The Call

Many of us are too busy or too afraid to step out of our daily lives and see things as they really are. We want to lose weight, but life gets in the way. We promise ourselves that someday we will be thin, but right now we can't find the time to lose weight. Instead, we bake cakes and cookies for church fund-raisers, scouting events, soccer teams, Little League, school parties, and first days at camp. We are too busy scheduling activities for our families and running from one appointment to another. We are too busy chairing committees and volunteering at organizations that feed the hungry. We promise ourselves that next week, perhaps, we will find the time to diet and go for a walk, but next week comes and there are even more chores to do, errands to run, problems to solve, and decisions to make. Dieting will have to wait.

We are too busy writing reports, arguing cases, saving patients' lives, creating new software companies, running corporations, and trading on Wall Street to find a moment to think about ourselves. At home we are busy trying to be the good spouses who whip up gourmet meals with two desserts. We are busy trying to be the wonderful parents who attend to the children's and grandchildren's every need. We spend our lives trying to be great at everything we do. We try to be even better than most because we must make up for the fact that we are fat and therefore worth less than thin people.

We learned this lesson very early in life and incorporate it into all that we do. Fat means lazy. Fat means dumb. Fat means undesirable. Fat means getting paid less, especially if you are a woman. Excessive weight is social suicide, instant death. No matter what we may have succeeded at in life, our weight cancels everything out and stands as our value to the world. Fat means settling for less.

We know this. We believe it and we accept it, and we let it go because it is the only way we can get on with our lives, but in our hearts we believe that one day we will be able to lose all of our weight. We even convince ourselves that our present suffering will be rewarded in that distant future when we are thin. Not only do we believe that we will be thin, we think that all that was lost in our lives will be regained. We will star in the leading role in the senior play, we will be voted prom queen, captain of the football team, or most likely to succeed. We will get that fantastic job, marry the right spouse, live happily ever after, and look great doing it. We tell ourselves this because it is the only way we can make it in a thin world—pretend that one day our dreams will come true. But we reach a point where we just can't swallow it anymore. Something inside us detonates. In that one crystalline moment we step out of our everyday lives and see ourselves as we really are, and it is a horrifying experience. We see our lives as cramped, contained, unfulfilled, and wasted. We see our fat as the entire description of our existence. It defines us, plagues us, and will eventually kill us. We see time passing us by. We see ourselves as mere observers in our own lives rather than participants in them. Anthropologists describe this realization moment as a crisis conversion. Ricers know it as the Call. It is that epiphany that moves us from our ordinary lives to extraordinary ones. The Call is what wakes us up and brings us to Durham.

When I began collecting interviews from Ricers, I started with those like me—people who were new to Durham and to the Rice Diet experience. I picked Carol Daly because I knew her to be funny, blunt, and knowledgeable about diet culture. Even though she had been in Durham only a short time, she seemed to be friends with just about everybody. She was popular, and if she enjoyed our interview experience, she would tell others, and I would have an easier time finding people willing to tell me their life stories. I also chose Carol because she was worshipped by all the men at the Rice House, and probably by men everywhere. She was obese like the rest of us, but that didn't seem to stop men of all ages from flocking around her. I wanted to know her secret.

The interview took place at Carol's rental home in Durham. Her house was a study in minimalism. The walls, carpeting, draperies, and furniture were all white; the only color in the room was Carol. She was stretched out on the sofa like some grand pasha in a peach satin caftan that enhanced her skin tones. The point of the design of the house was to focus all attention on her. It was effective. I couldn't take my eyes off her.

She motioned me to the only chair in the room, and I balanced my bag, tape recorder, and notebook on my lap while Carol relaxed even deeper into the couch. She reminded me of that Goya painting of the reclining nude. I was convinced that her posing was deliberate. As I turned on the tape recorder, a young woman appeared with a tray of oranges and Diet Rite soda—the drink of Ricers because of its low sodium content—and without a word set the tray on the floor in front of the couch. The woman left the room and I heard the front door shut. Carol peeled her orange slowly and began her tale.

Carol Daly

"When I was a little girl I was fatter than everyone else, but I never let that stand in my way. My mother put me on a diet when I was young, and it just didn't work. She tried to get me to follow the diet—it was Weight Watchers—but I just couldn't do it. I was tired and cranky and hungry all the time. One day she took me aside and said, 'Carol, you will never be thin and popular. You will have to develop a great personality so people will like you in spite of your weight.' So I did. I became adept at getting people to like me. I would practice staring them down when they looked at me. If somebody made a rude remark about my weight, I would give them a really sharp and witty retort. I took no crap off of anybody about my weight. I felt horrible inside, like something was really wrong with me, but I didn't let it show.

"I have lived all over the world but spent most of my time in Cairo. In Egypt, I didn't feel fat. They like bigger women, so really I felt like a princess there. In Europe and America, I was very self-conscious about my weight. Who wouldn't be? I much prefer the Middle East.

"I got the Call to Durham during sex. No kidding. I was in Cairo, Egypt, at the Ritz Hotel having sex with my boyfriend. We were in the bathtub—this big marble thing, really beautiful. Anyway, we were having sex, and I was on the bottom. After we were finished I tried to get up, but I was wedged in so tightly I just couldn't move. My boyfriend tried to pull me out but couldn't. After about an hour of struggling we finally gave up and realized we needed professional help. He called the front desk of the hotel and explained the situation to them. They sent up a couple of maintenance men to extract me from the tub. They were very nice and polite about this—after all, this was the Ritz. Still, I was mortified. The next day I called Durham and got Dr. Kempner's assistant. In two weeks, I was in Durham on the Rice Diet."

I heard noises upstairs. Carol looked toward the stairs and smiled. The interview was over. She dismissed me with a wave of her hand, heaved herself up from the couch, and went upstairs. I gathered my things and left. When I saw her the next morning at the Rice House she nodded to me from across the room, but didn't come over to speak. However, Vincent Petrella, a retired newspaperman, did. He had heard about the interview from Carol when he met her for a round of midnight bowling. I had had no idea that there was a Ricer bowling league!

Vincent just sat down at the table and began to recite his life story to me. Everyone at the surrounding tables stopped talking and looked at him. The whole Rice House was listening. I hurried to find my tape recorder. Vince didn't look at me or at others as he spoke, instead staring off into space.

Vincent Petrella

"I was a dying man. I had had three heart attacks and one quadruple-bypass surgery. I had done everything I could to get well. I wasn't fat, or at least I didn't think I was. I came to Duke, and they told me that I was a hundred pounds overweight, but I didn't even know it! I thought of myself as stocky, not fat. I am a strong man, too, not a weakling.

"I didn't think I was fat, but my heart did. I was suffocating. I was in the hospital with my last surgery and my whole family was praying for me. I had everyone I knew, my whole parish, praying, passing out saints' cards, holding healing services, the works. Anyway, my wife was driving home one night praying. When she got home, she turned on the television, and there was a doctor talking about the Rice Diet. They had someone on there whose life was saved by the Diet. The show went on about how going to Durham could save the dying and how people who other doctors had given up on were cured in Durham. My wife called the hospital and told me about it. I remember hearing the words 'Rice Diet' and I just perked up. It's as though a light went on.

"It was late at night, but my wife called the Rice Diet Clinic. She wasn't expecting anyone to answer; she thought she would get a recording—but someone did answer. She told them the desperateness of the situation. They booked me in at Duke, and I was there in three days.

"You know, the Rice Diet is closed at night. We asked around and never did find out who answered that phone. I knew it was divine intervention. That is why I am in Durham, and that is why I am alive today. It's a miracle."

The entire Rice House was silent, and then people began nodding their heads in agreement with the conviction that the Rice Diet truly does heal the sick. I had heard rumors of people who were near death from heart disease, diabetes, or some other horrible condition, only to be resurrected through the power of rice and fruit. Vincent showed me that those rumors were true.

After hearing Vincent's testimony, I went to Duke's east campus to walk the Wall. I wanted some stillness so I could absorb the meaning of the words I had just recorded. I walk the wall when I need to think, need some peace, or just need time alone. I also walk it after each meal. It is my way of acknowledging that even the small amount of food we receive at the Rice House must be balanced with a lot of exercise.

I met Elizabeth Grant on one of my ritual walks. Elizabeth, a physician from Australia, left her family, career, and country to lose weight in Durham. She wanted me to hear her story and to document her experience. I stopped and got my tape recorder out of my fanny pack. Elizabeth stood patiently as I found a blank tape. That was the last time she stopped moving during our entire interview. She walked at a fast pace, and I struggled to keep up.

I found it odd that a doctor would have such a difficult time with obesity. Doctors are always telling their overweight patients to lose the weight. Why couldn't Elizabeth follow her own advice? She explained to me that overeating and dieting were not knowledge based. All the knowledge in the world can't make you thin. She believed that the cause of obesity was a combination of factors and influences and may be too deeply imbedded to ferret out.

Elizabeth Grant

"It's weird how that happens. I am a doctor. I know about all the hazards of obesity. I tell my patients to lose weight, and they just look at me and think, 'Physician, heal thyself.' I had all the knowledge and have been on a ton of diets, but just couldn't do it. I left my job, husband, family, and patients to come to Durham. I've lost 130 pounds so far, and it is unbelievable. Just like that. For years I tried to lose weight and couldn't, and I come to Durham, and the weight flies off. It's just like magic.

"I was desperate to lose weight, and I couldn't find anything like the Rice Diet in Australia. There are lots of diet programs there, but nothing like the Rice House. I heard about the Rice Diet from a friend of mine's mother. She had gone to Durham years ago and lost a lot of weight. She's still fat, but she was once pretty thin. I went to my family doctor, and he told me that at my weight, the

Rice Diet was my only hope. Still, I didn't want to go to Durham, North Carolina. I had no idea what it would be like. I didn't want to leave home, leave my family.

"I was at a family picnic. It was a family reunion actually, and everybody was there. There were tables piled with food, and I was in the food line with my paper plate. I was on autopilot, just spooning food from the many dishes onto my plate. I went back to the table where my husband was and sat down. I couldn't fit at the picnic table because of my bulk, and I couldn't fit in a lawn chair because my hips and butt wouldn't squeeze into it. My husband would bring my own reinforced chair from home. You would think that would have humiliated me enough to lose weight, but no, no. I was sitting in my chair next to my cousin—she is thin and eats like a pig. She was talking to me and, all of a sudden, I couldn't hear her words and I knew I had to go to Durham *now*. Whatever it was inside me just exploded, and all those years of denial melted. I just got up and left. Six weeks later I was in Durham."

I was fascinated and a bit disappointed that Elizabeth, a doctor, would have the same struggles with weight as everyone else. I'd hoped that she would be privy to some medical insight that could change her behavior or that she would know of some cure. She just insisted that knowledge had nothing to do with insight. She needed the power of the Call to change her destructive behavior. She, like all of us, needed Durham and the Rice Diet.

I was surprised to find another doctor on the Rice Diet. Sally Standoff, a retired pediatrician from Florida, came to my aid during a crisis. I was living in Chapel Hill and attending graduate school when I was mugged on a city bus while coming home after a class. To make matters worse, the mugger lived in the apartment building right next to mine. I was afraid to stay at my apartment that night and didn't have any place to go on such short notice. Sally, whom I had never spoken to at the Rice House, heard me tell others of my situation and offered to let me stay with her in her apartment until I found another place to live.

I knew Sally was on the Rice Diet because I saw her at meals, but I found her a bit standoffish because she never walked with us, went to movies, or participated in other Ricer events. She kept pretty much to herself and would come early to each meal, eat her bowl of rice, and take her two fruits with her. She didn't show up for meals on weekends. Of all the people at the Rice House, I would have expected Sally to be the last one to help me out.

I went with her to her place after dinner. Sally told me that she would cure me of my fear of going back to my apartment and that I would never be afraid again. She told me that she wasn't afraid of anything, that nothing could scare her. I believed her. That night, in the living room of her rental apartment, she pulled a gun from her fanny pack and placed it in my trembling hand. For the next couple of hours, I learned to load and unload that pistol—even in the dark. To this day, I can still do it. I learned how to flick it back into firing position with a snap of my wrist. I was really getting the hang of it! That night, after Sally had gone to sleep, I lay in the twin bed across the room from hers. I wondered if I had to get up to use the bathroom in the middle of the night, would Sally mistake me for a burglar and plug me with one of the several loaded weapons she had stashed throughout the apartment? I could see the headlines in the Durham *Herald-Sun:* "Ricer killed in a lover's quarrel." "Starving Ricer goes berserk and murders one of her own." I didn't make a move all night long. I even breathed as quietly as I could.

The next morning, after a breakfast of oatmeal at the Rice House, we drove to a shooting range near Raleigh, and I spent Easter Sunday shooting round after round, first with a twenty-two and later with a Glock nine millimeter. In the beginning I missed the target entirely, but later I got inside one of the rings, and finally I got two kill shots right through the paper head. Sally was wrong. I was more afraid than ever. My hands shook and my heart raced every time I pulled the trigger. She said I would get used to it; people can get used to anything.

On the drive back to Durham, Sally allowed me to turn on the tape recorder. She proceeded to tell me of her Call to the Rice Diet and what brought her to Durham. My ears were still ringing from the noise at the shooting range, and Sally's voice sounded muffled as she began.

Sally Stanhoff

"I had always known about the Rice Diet and Durham. I mean, when you are in the medical profession, you just know that the Rice Diet is where the nearly dead end up. I knew about it for the treatment of kidney disease.

"When I got married, I tried to have a baby, but I kept miscarrying. I would miscarry right at the end of the first trimester. Well, I just started to put on weight. Before, when things would upset me I would worry so much I'd forget to eat. I would just miss meals. Then things changed. I just started to be hungry all the time, ravenously hungry. I would watch the clock to see if it was time to eat yet. Before, when I got scared or nervous or upset, I couldn't eat; I wouldn't be able to swallow. Then all of a sudden I couldn't stop swallowing. I was so self-conscious that I wouldn't eat anything in front of people. Of course, I wouldn't even make it home to eat. I would starve through a business luncheon and drive through McDonald's on the way home. I would stop at a gas station and dispose of the evidence before I got home. It took longer to get that stale grease smell out of the car. I would use Joy perfume. I'd sprinkle it on the car seats. I didn't want my husband to know that I stopped at McDonald's. I was supposed to be dieting. He nagged me constantly about weight. Kids sniggered at me in the grocery store. I took it. Now I wouldn't, but then I did. People, mere acquaintances, would tell me that I would look so much better if I lost weight. No kidding!

"I divorced my husband. I just looked up at him one day and said, 'That's it. No more.' I couldn't stand it. It was a nasty, nasty divorce. My second husband was my childhood sweetheart. He was the man I was supposed to marry in the first place. He didn't care if I was fat or thin. We got married twenty minutes after my divorce from my first husband became final. Then one day on the tennis court, he just keeled over dead with a massive heart attack. There was no warning; nothing. That was it. He wasn't even fat. I had to go through all of his papers, and that's when I found out I was essentially broke. The finances were in a shambles. He owed everybody money. I buried him with the $255 you get from Social Security when somebody dies. That was all the money I had. The bank foreclosed on my house. I lost the car. His children deserted me, my friends wouldn't return my calls, and I had to move in with my sister. It was all very humiliating.

"That's when I decided to become a doctor. I wanted a profession where I could make a living and take care of myself. I gained even more weight in school. I had no time to eat right or exercise. I had no social life and didn't want one. All I did was study.

"One holiday, I think it was Easter, I took a trip to St. Thomas with my sister and her family. I was sitting on the plane next to my sister and another lady when the stewardess came by and said, 'There is an empty seat at the back of the plane in case your daughter wants more room.' I don't know what stunned me more—the fact that the stewardess thought I was old enough to be my sister's mother or that I was so fat she just assumed my sister didn't have enough room in the seat next to mine. I had a magazine open on my lap, and there was an article on the Rice Diet. Something clicked, and I remembered reading about the Rice Diet before. I liked the idea of it: all white food, all pure. I was on the next plane to Durham."

When we got back to her apartment we didn't speak much. I guess she'd told me more about herself than she had intended. It made her vulnerable, and she didn't like feeling that way. She preferred to be the one in control. I gathered my things, thanked her, and left. It was early evening as I walked up Cardiac Hill to the Rice House, sat on the porch for a while and thought of Sally, her arsenal, and her hard life.

Most people who come to Durham to diet keep coming back. It is the only way to keep off the weight. In Durham the focus of one's existence is diet and exercise. Once we are home, different priorities arise. I was very interested in repeaters because they represented the elders of diet culture. They knew all about dieting, how to get the weight off fast, and more importantly, how to keep it off.

Paul Porter, the chief executive officer of an international telecommunications company, was the first repeater who agreed to be interviewed, and then only after I pestered him about it for a couple of weeks. Paul relented on the condition that he direct—or rather dominate—the entire interview process. He wanted to meet at the bar of the Washington Duke Inn. He would speak and I would listen. I agreed to his demands and immediately regretted it. I thought the interview would be hostile and basically useless, but I had never been to the Washington Duke, and I wanted to experience its luxury.

That evening, I scanned the parking lot of the hotel looking for Paul's car. People told me that he was very rich. I made sure to park my twelve-year-old orange Toyota Tercel next to Paul's customized, hand-finished Jaguar.

He was standing at the bar, and he tapped his watch when he looked up and saw me. I wasn't late. He was just asserting his authority through impatience. I deliberately took my time setting up my tape recorder, gathering my paper, selecting the proper pen for the occasion. As Paul was scolding me for my slowness, a waiter brought me a glass of wine, a Merlot, and later came by with the bottle. I prefer red wines to white, and I particularly like a thick red. Paul had no way of knowing this, and I was thrown a little off balance. Fifteen minutes later, a waitress brought us dinner. Paul had taken care of everything. Initially, I was flattered. He wanted this to be a nice evening, and he cared enough to order wine and dinner. I was touched by his generosity and began to relax. Later, I realized that he behaved this way with everyone, and my defenses went back up to their natural position. When he was ready, I pressed the record button of my tape recorder.

Paul Porter

"Okay, I had no choices in life. Let's get that straight from the start. I didn't wake up rich. I worked my way up, worked the American Dream. I was so poor most of my life, especially growing up. I wanted to have a different life. I wanted to be a naval officer and go to Annapolis. I knew that was a long shot because I was a short, fat, poor kid. I figured out the only way a poor kid can make it in this world is to find a need and fill it. It's the oldest thing in the world and the easiest. People are basically lazy, and they will pay someone to do the chores they don't want to do. So I did those chores. And then I'd hire others to do them for me, and soon I had my own company at sixteen. I made a lot of money, and I had fingers in many pots. I knew that telecommunications was it for the future, so I decided that that was what I was going to do. I joined the Army. That was the only service that would let a fat boy like me in, with my poor eyesight. The Army takes everybody. I did my time and then got out and went to school with my G. I. benefits. I had studied communications while I was in school. Made a fortune, bought and sold several companies and was successful in every sense of the word. Had a beautiful wife. I've had several now, but they were all beautiful. Nice successful kids—I was living the good life. Everything was going fine and then one day, I was driving down the highway, down the L. A. Freeway. I got this intense pressure in my ribs. It felt as though someone was hammering on my chest. I pulled off the road and was gasping for breath. I used the car phone to dial 911, and I woke up with tubes and everything sticking out of me and the word Durham in my head. No kidding—I saw Durham as if someone had written it on my retinas. Four weeks later I was in Durham on the Rice Diet. I come back four times a year. It's the coming back to Durham that keeps me alive."

Paul leaned back in his chair and the interview part of our evening was over. He asked me to turn off the tape recorder and put down my pen. We left the dining room to have coffee and cordials by the fire. We didn't speak much. Instead, we sank deeper into the soft cushions of the overstuffed chairs as the warmth from the fire and the alcohol took their toll. I dozed off, and when I awoke Paul was gone and my glass had been refilled.

Abby Felcher is also a repeater. She comes to Durham each time she starts gaining weight. A divorced, middle-aged attorney from New York City, she is funny, straightforward, and honest. Abby has been to the Rice House four times and considers herself an expert on the Diet. She is a mother and a grandmother, but nevertheless is slim and stylish. She always wears designer clothes and is an avid reader of fashion magazines.

I never thought of myself as particularly unfashionable until I met Abby; she was always trying to correct my wardrobe. For a year after our initial interview, she would send me magazine clippings and articles on clothes and makeup in the hope that I would heed her advice. She would often tell me to push up the sleeves of my shirt, and to this day I do it because I remember her informing me that I would look better if I did. It's funny—this advice coming from almost anyone else would have angered me or hurt my feelings, but somehow Abby just made me feel as if I were being taken care of.

For the first interview, I met Abby at her condo. It was as neat and fashionable as the woman herself; the carpet and walls were beige, and she'd hung framed primary-color prints. I marveled secretly at her housekeeping abilities and resolved to be neater myself. We sat down to herbal tea and apple-flavored rice crackers—Abby's idea of cheating on the Diet—and she began.

Abby Felcher

"I was the typical American housewife, I guess, except I had my own successful business. My husband and I were both professionals. I started out in the early 1960s with my own practice, and that was practically unheard of then. Anyway, I had never been what you would call fat. I was sort of chubby at times. I would gain weight as a teenager and get depressed because people treat you like crap when you put on weight, but then I would go on a diet and lose it and feel good again. I was thin by sheer willpower in young adulthood. Then one day my husband said I looked matronly. I thought, no kidding. Here I am almost fifty years old and have two grown children and three grandchildren and so what if I have put on a little padding? Still, what he had said to me sank in, so I joined Weight Watchers. Lived off cans of tuna packed in water and one glass of wine a day. When we went out to dinner, I would have three ounces of grilled meat which I would pat dry with the napkin, a half-cup of cottage cheese, and one peach half. My husband would sit across from me and knock back two or three Beefeaters and a fifteen-ounce prime rib, and lecture me on my inability to lose weight. I would sit there just hoping he would keel over with a massive heart attack. Then, out of the blue, my husband moved out and filed for divorce. He sued me for half the property and half of my practice! I looked in the mirror and said to myself, 'You're going to Durham.'

"I had heard about Durham from the ex-governor of New Jersey's wife, Betty Hughes, who wrote an article in the *Ladies' Home Journal*. I still have that article. Also, a friend of mine had gone to Durham and lost a lot of weight. I was almost a hundred pounds overweight by then. I couldn't believe it, but I was. I felt so guilty about it, so bad and useless. It's as though when I looked in the mirror I really saw myself as others saw me, and it was horrible, horrible! I sold the practice, settled with my ex, rented my home, told the kids goodbye, got in the car, and drove to Durham.

"The first time I was here I stayed approximately four months. Had a great time. Loved every minute of it. I lost fifty-two pounds. I would have stayed longer and gotten to goal weight, but I couldn't because one of my daughters became ill. She was diagnosed with breast cancer. I had to go home to be with her and help with the grandchildren. At home, with all of the stress and sorrow, the weight just came back on. I didn't have time to eat diet meals, or exercise. I was too busy running to doctors' appointments and chemotherapy sessions. She would have a series of chemo treatments and get really ill. Sometimes they would have to hospitalize her, and I would sit in the waiting room and live out of vending machines. When she died, I forced myself to get involved with groups and social activities. I stayed busy, but I just didn't have anything left to give. I had lost Cathy, my daughter, young in life, and we were very close. It was a stupid way for her to die, I thought. Cancer: I should have gotten it, I am the parent. It is not right that your child precede you in death. It is not natural.

"Anyway, I wasn't conscious of overeating, but I blew up fast. Gained over a hundred pounds. Still, I didn't want to come back to Durham because everyone would see that I'd gained the weight back, and I wanted to be one of the few that actually made it, actually kept their weight off. I went to all kinds of health resorts and spas: Golden Door, Pritikin, Hempstead Heath in England, even that secret place in Florida. Didn't make any difference. One afternoon I was sitting in this group of women at a Weight Watchers meeting. I had joined yet again. I looked around at everyone and said out loud, 'I am going to Durham.' I got up and left.

"The second time in Durham, I almost made it to goal weight, came within fifteen pounds. I had plastic surgery on my body and a facelift. I exercised constantly and walked sixteen miles a day. All I did was walk all over Durham. I bought a bikini and looked good in it too. Had a total makeover. Bought a Porsche. Changed my entire life. Now I return to Durham as soon as I gain ten pounds. That's the only way."

There are some dieters who find Durham so crucial to their weight loss that they never leave. Instead, they make a home for themselves in Durham and continue to diet.

The first person I interviewed who came to Durham to diet and stayed was Sarah Jacobs. Sarah is a petite forty-five-year-old businesswoman who owns a chain of nationally known retail stores.

I was anxious about interviewing Sarah because I didn't know her well. She was what I considered an old-line Ricer: she had been on the Rice Diet a very long time and was one of the chosen few who was close to the Rice Diet doctors. She was pleasant but not friendly, forthcoming when prompted but not open. Also, she was very thin, and I was not. I felt clumsy and awkward around her. I was still struggling to get to goal weight, while Sarah had reached nirvana. She was where I wanted to be, but didn't believe that I could actually get there—not in this lifetime.

We met at the Rice House for the interview, but the dining room was still noisy with Ricers gabbing and vying for the last morsel of rice, so we walked to Sarah's home instead. Her home, four short blocks from the Rice House, was tiny. The three front rooms looked like something that a monk or cloistered nun would inhabit. There was not a hint of luxury or even comfort. No television, radio, CD player, or phone that I could see. As I looked around for a place to set up my recorder, Sarah began her story.

Sarah Jacobs

"I got the Call at my sweet sixteen birthday party—except it wasn't so sweet.

"Actually it was my mother who received the Call. She decided I was too fat and I needed to do something about it, and fast. Looking back at the pictures from that time, I wasn't even fat, just chunky. It was the time of Twiggy, and everybody was expected to be perfect. Children were especially required to be perfect, and that meant thin and pretty with long straight hair. That wasn't me. My parents and my whole family were always freaking about my weight. It was the constant chant at the dinner table. 'Sarah, don't eat that. Sarah, use some self-control. Sarah, you must lose weight.' My sister is thin. Both my parents are thin. Nobody could figure out why I was fat. My home life was difficult because the nagging about weight was relentless. You know, let's pick on the fat kid so we don't have to look at the fact that we are one big dysfunctional family. 'If only Sarah were thin, we would all be happy.' My parents would say that stuff to their friends all the time with me standing there. So I came to Durham.

"I adored Durham. I didn't lose any weight, but I had a great time. So great, in fact, that the doctors phoned my parents and said, 'Come and get this kid, she is not dieting and is having too good a time here.' So my parents came and got me. Back home, I couldn't wait to get back to Durham. I missed it so. Instead, my parents sent me to fat camps in the Catskills. There I was supervised but didn't lose much weight, and it wasn't any fun like Durham.

"Back in the city I was on Weight Watchers, which I hated. My food and activity were constantly monitored by my mother. I couldn't eat what the other kids ate. I hated my life. The second time I came to Durham, I got the Call myself. I was hanging out with my friends and they were talking about some inane teenage stuff, and I just knew that I didn't belong there, I belonged in Durham. I went home and said, 'Take me back to Durham.' They did. Drove straight down 95. Took twelve hours, but I was home in Durham. I stayed four months and got really thin. My parents came to get me at the end of my stay and were so proud. They were happy with each other for a while, and maybe it was because I was thin.

"I stayed away from the Rice House for almost a decade. I got fat again. Kept it off for over a decade, and then the magic wore off. One Christmas I was at my cousin's house in Long Island, and we were all eating and drinking and I saw my reflection in the mirror across from the dining room table. I was totally taken aback. My body looked as if it was melting into the chair I was sitting on. I was just this mass of flesh, a blob with a head. I heard a voice inside me say 'Durham.' That was it. I now live in Durham permanently."

When I left Sarah, she picked up her journal and began to write. I walked back to the Rice House, amazed that anyone could be so dedicated to dieting and thinness that they could become an ascetic like Sarah. No wonder she was so thin. Her whole life was devoted to it. More power to her. I shuddered and knew I could never adhere to the Diet that diligently and would never be that thin.

Tom Brooks is another Ricer who came to Durham to lose weight and never left. Unlike Sarah, Tom is not an ascetic, but a repeater—perhaps because he has too much going on in his life to devote all of his time and energy to the Diet. An attorney, novelist and new father, he is an ex-Chicagoan who considers Durham home.

I met Tom at the Ninth Street Bakery (now Elmo's Diner) for the interview. As usual, the place was packed with Ricers, students, professors, and street people. Normally it would have been very difficult to record someone's voice over the din of the dining room, but Tom was loud and boisterous by nature, and I had no trouble distinguishing his remarks from the comments of people around us on the tape. The whole Bakery laughed along with me at Tom's witticisms. He presented a great life story and was delighted to share it with everyone within hearing distance. All he needed was a good audience, and I suspect he never encountered a bad one.

To many people, Tom's story would seem shtick, something you would hear on late-night television. To me, it was performance, and I loved it. Tom leaned his massive body back and propped a foot up on an adjacent chair, pulled out a cigar despite the smoking restriction sign near the door, and began his tale.

Tom Brooks

"The first time I came here was twenty years ago. I, well, I just reached a point where I was disgusted with myself. It was my birthday. Seventeen years old and really fat. I was a fat kid most of my life. I got thinner when my parents sent me to the fat camps, Camp Stanley in the Catskills. I will never forget that. I always returned to fat when I got back home.

"At my birthday party, all of my friends and my friends' parents were there. My mom had ordered the whole party catered. There was all this food and I wanted it, but I was very conscious that I was fat and all eyes were on what I was eating. Right then and there I decided to come to Durham. Didn't finish my junior year in high school. Instead, I spent it in Durham. I had heard about the Rice Diet forever. Friends of my parents had gone. A fat cousin had gone, that sort of thing. I just got in the car and drove to Durham all by myself. My parents had fixed it up with the Rice House that I was coming, and they called the Holiday Inn and booked me a room. The Holiday Inn was the place to be the first time I was in Durham. It was rocking. Durham was all sex, drugs, and rock and roll then, and I loved every minute of it. I lost all of my weight just like that. It was the quick fix I needed. I lost thirty-five pounds the first month. I came to Durham fat and went home thin. Just like that.

"I was really thin for the first time. I looked so good. I bought these tiny jeans and tight running shorts. I had the flattest stomach. I felt invincible. Women loved me. Girls that used to make fun of me called me up for dates. Everybody wanted to have sex with me. Unbelievable. I was like an Adonis.

"The effect of Durham lasted about a month. For the first month I had no problems, but I wasn't prepared for the outside world and the incredible eating pressures at home. Let's face, it at home you are constantly feeding. That's what I call it. Home is a feeding trough. I am a food sociopath. If I am around people who are eating like pigs, then I too will eat like a pig and think nothing of it. I will have no twinge of guilt. I will eat what is put in front of me. At the Rice House, all that was put in front of me was rice and fruit. On the drive back home I gained twenty pounds plus. Once home I did everything in the world not to come back to Durham. I went to Pritikin in California. I went to behavior modification classes, Weight Watchers, Overeaters Anonymous—the whole nine yards. I went to spas and did all the diets. All the main ones plus the minor ones. Nothing equals Durham. I kept saying to myself, tomorrow I will go back to Durham. I didn't want to go back. Didn't want to admit that I was a failure, that I couldn't handle the outside world. Still, I knew deep down that I had to go back. Then a few weeks ago I had my physical and found out that I was diabetic and would have to go on insulin. I thought that's it, that's it and no more. It's Durham or die. I didn't want to die, so I came back to the Rice House. I will never leave Durham again."

The interview ended abruptly when Tom's very thin wife walked in. She had a chilling effect on him. Immediately, he sat up straight, put out his cigar, and became very formal. She sat down at our table and we chatted a few minutes. He thanked me for the interview and paid the bill. Then they left. I was amazed by the rapid change in Tom's behavior and wondered what he was like at home: the wild funny guy or the quiet, subdued attorney at law.

David Blum also lives in Durham. I met him at a coffee shop within walking distance of the Rice House. David is one of those people who have no visible means of support but live very well. He told me that he was semiretired and once owned a manufacturing company that has now gone public. He announced to me at our first meeting that he had been married at least four times and has children by all of his wives and some of his girlfriends. In fact, he was the father of an entire tribe. He stated these statistics proudly and in a booming voice that was heard by everyone in the coffee shop. The people around us looked our way and leaned forward so they could hear better. I was impressed by his productivity and told him so.

He, like Tom Brooks, needed an audience for his story. He came alive in the presence of others. He needed us to witness his story, to make sense of it. David began belligerently to lay out the facts of his life.

David Blum

"I'm fat. I know it. So what? I've known it all of my life. I was a chubby little fellow. I was short and fat but wouldn't take any crap off of anybody. Other kids were afraid of me. I was so angry most of the time. I would clobber somebody if they said anything rude about my weight. I was always getting into fights. I didn't let it get me down. I had a chip on my shoulder. I played football in high school even though I was short—I was big and fast so I played.

"I knew about Durham forever. It's just around like some sort of secret society. I knew eventually I would get fat enough to qualify—and I did. First time I came here was when I was forty years old. It was my birthday. I was forty years old and in very bad shape physically. I had cellulitis, edema, swelling all over the place, sleep apnea, and I was only getting about forty-five percent of the oxygen I needed. My lungs were shutting down. Still, I kept on working. Had a phone to my ear the whole time. Business is so demanding that I was afraid that if I stopped for a moment the whole thing would collapse. I was forty years old, I couldn't get my trousers off due to the swelling in my legs and click—I was going to Durham. I had enough of the fat, and I was going to go to Durham and get it off even if they had to cut it out of me. I thought about Pritikin, but I knew he was a follower of Kempner, so I decided on Durham. I had my secretary find out about Durham and get me into something because I couldn't stand it anymore, couldn't stand my life. The next thing I knew she had booked me into DFC [the Duke Diet and Fitness Center]. She took care of everything.

"I lost a ton of weight there. I was so big that I flunked the stress test, and they had me exercising at CFL [the Center For Living]. I switched to CFL and extended my stay in Durham by a couple of months. I didn't want to go home. Found my true home in Durham.

"When it was time to go back home, I thought I would prepare myself so I took all of these classes: nutrition, behavior modification, stress management, grocery store shopping, restaurant eating, the whole bit. I was armed with the knowledge I needed to maintain and perhaps continue my weight loss at home. I went back home, and everybody was knocked out by how I looked.

They couldn't believe it. Also, I was much nicer. Nothing bothered me. The stock market would drop three hundred points. Big deal. One of our trucks crashed and a hundred orders were lost. Never mind. Any time anything bothered me I would go for a walk. Soon, I was walking all the time. I was out of the office so much people assumed I had gone back to Durham.

"Home was a different thing than Durham. Home was a blast furnace. I went home, and it was as though I opened the door to Hell. All of these problems just engulfed me, and it was horrible. You know how it is. You walk in, and you know that you will be incinerated. Nothing has changed and it is hot as it ever was, and quickly you just go back to the old ways of reacting. That's what happened to me. People were yelling at me at work and at home and all I could hear roaring in my ears was the word Durham over and over. I went back to Durham and stayed ten months.

"I lost 150 pounds the second time around and looked and felt terrific. I stopped to smell the roses. Took up painting. Took up golf. Went to concerts and lecture series at Duke University. Took gardening classes. Did things I never even thought of. Had a wonderful time. Of course, my family was mad as hell that I was in Durham spending all of their supposed inheritance, but hey, I didn't care. I was loving life for the first time.

"Eventually, I had to go back home to my son's wedding. I didn't want to go, but I went anyway. Same old thing happened. I just got involved in the whole situation—the problems with the business, the problems at home. I promised myself that I wouldn't let it happen again—that I wouldn't get fat. For about six years I did really well. I would walk every morning and every evening. I played racquetball. I lifted weights. I took up yoga and meditation. I was very Zen. I would order a fruit plate wherever I went. Then one day, out of the blue, I ordered an Italian sub for lunch. One with sausage and peppers (red and green) and olive oil and cheese, and while you're at it how about a bag of chips and a Coke, a real one too, not a diet. I just went to hell from that day on, and I had this out-of-body experience. I saw myself looking down at me at my desk with a phone in both ears and a donut in each hand. I knew I had to go back to Durham.

"I got very, very ill. I was hospitalized. They thought I'd had a stroke, but they weren't sure. They called it a cerebral incident. I think it was an anxiety attack. My third wife came to the hospital with her lawyer—both teary-eyed. They assumed I was going to die. My wife pleaded with me to split the property with her; give her the share of the business. She told me that if I died she wouldn't even have a car to drive to my funeral. I said, 'Take a fucking cab!' That's it. Right then and there I got the Call to go back to Durham. Went to the Rice House and stayed. I live here now."

After hours of taping, I told David that I just had to go home. I was exhausted. He thanked me for interviewing him and, with a twinkle in his eye, told me, "If you play your cards right, you might be able to rate as wife number five, or six. Only time will tell." I appreciated the gesture and told him so. I took no offense. I knew for a fact that he told every woman at the Rice House the same thing. He was just a lonely man who really needed women around him. I kissed him when I left, and he squeezed my hand. On the way to my car, I mused that wife number five was out there somewhere and probably on the Rice Diet.

When I started collecting life stories, I had no idea what I would discover. What I found was that all of us had similar dieting histories. All of us had a Call epiphany—that moment when the light bulb clicked on in our heads and we realized that we were no longer going to live our fat lives or diet haphazardly. Instead, we were going to fight our obesity head-on. That moment calls us to Durham; the Journey takes us there.

four

The Journey to Durham

The Journey to Durham is the response to the Call. The motivation to get to the Rice House is a powerful one for the potential Ricer and involves personal sacrifice. The Ricer-in-the-making becomes an ascetic, a pilgrim on the road to Durham. The Journey to Durham brings us out of our everyday lives and unites us with a community of believers. In her book *The Rice Diet Report,* Ricer Judy Moscovitz describes the life changes she had to make in order to come to Durham:

> I resolved to put everything else aside and make this diet my priority. It was so important to me that I sold everything I owned to get the money I needed to go to Durham for a lengthy stay. I put my house on the market and sold all of my furniture. By the time I finished, not one book, not one picture, not one record remained.[19]

Judy left her home country, Canada, to come to the Rice House. She gave up her profession and left her family and friends for the chance to lose weight in Durham. Her story is typical of Ricers' determination to afford the Rice House. Dr. Kempner used to inform dieters—and now Dr. Rosati does—that no sacrifice is too great for the privilege of being on the Rice Diet and losing weight. The physical and social benefits are phenomenal, and no amount of money spent or time lost is to stand in the way of true health and cultural acceptance. Dr. Kempner told us to rob a bank if necessary to finance our dieting costs. Many of us sell our homes or get second mortgages in order to finance our time in Durham.

The Journey stage represents a period of joyful determination. The anxiety of coming to Durham is over; the decision has been made. We believe that a life of obesity and social rejection is soon to become a part of history, and a new life filled with love, success, and eternal happiness awaits us. The Journey begins when we receive the Call and concludes with our first meal in the Rice House. It is a Mardi Gras celebration before the Lenten fast of the Rice Diet begins.

The language used by Ricers to describe the Journey reflects religious themes. Food is spoken of as being "divine," pleasurable," "powerful," and "mysterious." Ricers have an intense involvement with food. We know that soon, when we begin the Rice Diet, this involvement must end. All of us know that the Rice Diet is very strict and has meager fare, so before we actually begin the Diet we have one last ritualistic fling with food. Ricers call this the Last Supper. This event involves consuming delicious foods that the Rice Diet will soon forbid. Since the average stay in Durham is three months, a dieter will eat large quantities of food in the hope that it will be enough to fill the void for a long, long time.

For many of us, pizza is the dominant food for Last Suppers. It contains all the things considered off-limits for life by the Rice Diet: cheese, salt, fat, and flavor. An early morning walk around Duke Towers (an apartment complex on Trinity Avenue where dieters rent by the week) reveals piles of Domino's Pizza boxes by the apartments' doors—each one a testament to the Rice Diet's strictness and dieters' longings for food.

The Journey, like the Call, differs initially along gender lines. Of the Ricers I talked with, women spoke first of leaving loved ones and family behind. Even single women without children worried about leaving parents, siblings, and close friends. Only later did women discuss the difficulty of leaving their professions and the problems associated with a long absence from their jobs. Women missed the closeness of relationships—how would their families get along without them? Who would take care of their children?

Men, on the other hand, worried primarily about lost time on the job, the progress of their competitors, and their ability to provide for their families.

Sharon Anderson, a public relations executive and a true believer in the power of positive thinking, knew that God had brought her to Durham. She pulled her chair close to mine at dinner one night and confided this to me. I nodded, and she continued to speak, glad to tell someone her story. Her small, breathless voice was hard to hear above the din of the Rice House dining room, so we agreed to meet later at the bar at the Sheraton. That too was noisy, crowded, and full of smoke. My eyes stung and my throat burned as I struggled to hear Sharon's voice among all those shouting for attention. She leaned over and screamed into my tape recorder as she began her story.

Sharon Anderson

"Let me say this right up front. I believe that there are no insignificant acts in life and that coming to Durham is the most important and powerful event that has ever happened to me. I have been married, have two children, and got a divorce, but all of that pales next to the decision to come to the Rice House.

"I had decided to come to Durham a long time ago. I made the commitment to myself in my heart. You know when you promise yourself you will do something wonderful in your life? Some people want to scale Mount Everest or swim the Barrier Reef. My dream was to go to the Rice House, lose all of my weight, and live the life I was supposed to live. I was worried about leaving my family because they are very dependent on me. How would they function without me? I was concerned about my job. Would I get fired? Would they replace me? When I told my family I was going to Durham, they were thrilled. When I told my boss he said, 'Hurrah!' and gave me six months off with pay. Once I decided to go to Durham, everything fell into place. It was as though God opened that door for me.

"I loved the anticipation I felt getting ready for the big adventure. I went to the best salon in town and got a total makeover. Had a deep tissue massage. It was the first time I'd had a massage. I was always too embarrassed to get one before, but hey, I was going to Durham, and I wanted to be at my best. They had a big blowout party for me at work. Naturally, there was a ton of food there. People just don't get it, do they? My family had a big party with even more food. It was quite lovely, but I didn't want the fuss.

"My boyfriend went with me as far as D.C. We spent the weekend at the Four Seasons Hotel in Georgetown. We lived off room service, had mimosas and eggs Benedict for breakfast. I was trying to get in all the best meals before the Rice Diet. I used to take *Gourmet* magazine and drool over the pictures. I am a really good cook and would have these big dinner parties where I did all the cooking. I would always go to new restaurant openings. I would miss all of that on the Rice Diet.

"I met a guy at the Rice House who told me that he planned to commit suicide, but he was afraid he would miss some new snack product coming out. Said Combos saved him last time. He loved Combos [little pretzel tubes stuffed with flavored fillings] and if it hadn't been for them he would have ended his life. I know that sounds extremely weird, but I also know how he feels.

"My boyfriend and I ate all weekend in D.C. We ate Mexican food, Italian food, French food, Ben & Jerry's ice cream by the quart—everything I wanted. It was like heaven to have all of that food. You can get everything delivered to your room in D.C.—fabulous food from quality restaurants. After that weekend I put him on a plane home and continued the drive down to Durham. At South Hill, Virginia I had the last binge. South Hill is the final stop before you enter North Carolina. I don't eat off-program once I cross the state line, so South Hill is my last goodbye to food for a long time. In South Hill, the first time I came down, I ate at McDonald's, Kentucky Fried Chicken, and Pizza Hut. I stayed all afternoon, and it got late so I stayed overnight at the Holiday Inn. I didn't tell anyone because my friends and family would have been mortified. My boyfriend probably wouldn't have understood why I wanted junk food when I had just eaten fine food with him. The next morning I got up and had a sausage biscuit for breakfast from McDonald's and drove on in to Durham later that day."

Sharon finished her story and pulled out a bag of shredded wheat squares, which she always carried with her. She parceled out eleven squares for me and eleven for herself. We ordered another round of seltzer water, and I felt happy and relieved, as though a burden had been lifted from me. Perhaps Sharon was right. All things were possible, even reaching my goal weight. All I had to do was follow the Rice Diet and believe. We must all believe in the power of the Rice Diet, or we wouldn't be here in Durham following it.

If Sharon was a believer in positive thinking, Sylvia Goldman was the proof of its power. I interviewed Sylvia at her apartment at Duke Towers. She was very thin and like Abby Felcher and many other Ricers I have known, considered herself well versed in all things stylish and fashionable. For the interview, she wore black silk pajamas and a red jacket. I wore jeans, a sweater that another Ricer had given me, and tennis shoes. Again, like Abby, Sylvia took it upon herself to improve my appearance. She critiqued me from head to toe and took notes as she observed my fashion failures. Later, after I had gotten to know her better, Sylvia and her friends took me shopping and helped me find a more suitable wardrobe.

Her apartment was like every other rental at Duke Towers and consisted of a bedroom, living room, bath, and kitchen, but everywhere there were piles and piles of clothes. Sylvia collected clothes like some people collect antiques, and she often bought several colors of the same item. She told me that she could go three weeks without repeating an outfit. I gathered up a stack of cashmere sweaters from the sofa and breathed in the scent of them. Carefully placing them on the floor, I sat on the sofa and arranged my things. Sylvia brought us cups of Red Zinger tea and began her story.

Sylvia Goldman

"Coming east from California I didn't have the luxury of the South Hill, Virginia Last Supper ritual. I didn't even go out to any special place to eat because I had been to them all already. I haven't cooked or had a meal at home in probably a decade. We eat out all the time. We go to a lot of functions so there is no point in cooking at home. I never have food in the house anyway, because I am always on a diet. I do have this pre-Rice Diet ritual though. I eat a box of goldfish crackers and drink three martinis. That's my Last Supper. I also make a long list of food I am giving up for the Diet and what it means to me. One of the diet counselors I went to suggested this, and now I just incorporate it in any pre-Rice House visit. It is a stepping stone for me and gets me focused on the task ahead. I put all ethnic food on the list, as well as all salty food, because salt is strictly forbidden on the Rice Diet and it is what I miss the most. I love all kinds of chips and crackers. I love rice crackers, but even the fat-free ones will put weight on you. I am not a sweets person, so I don't miss any of that, but I do miss my martinis and my crackers.

"When I decided to come to Durham the first time, I was happy but a little afraid. I wasn't sure what I would encounter. I brought my whole family with me to give me some support. After a couple of days, I wanted everybody to go home because I was having such a good time. Before I left California, I sold the business because I didn't want anything to distract me from my weight loss. This was it for me. I wasn't getting any younger, and I knew that health problems would be catching up with me. I wanted to just stop the degeneration of my body. People thought I was nuts to just get up and go to Durham. My friends and business acquaintances couldn't understand what I was doing. After all, to them, I was just a chubby old woman who was foolish for going to Durham to lose weight. I didn't care. I simply didn't care what people thought. I had had enough of the weight. I had my Last Supper on American Airlines!"

A couple days after the interview, I got a call from Sylvia's personal stylist who insisted we meet for a consultation about my hair. Apparently Sylvia had been quite alarmed by my unflattering hairstyle and had arranged for her stylist to rescue me from my horribly unfashionable state. I went to his shop and allowed him to cut my hair very short and close to my head. He highlighted the parts that framed my face, and I left his shop $110 poorer and looking like a Palm Beach matron. I felt great. Now all I needed was the lifestyle to go with it.

Cindy Sitco was the next person I interviewed. We had a lot in common. She was single and about my age and weight. Like me, she was from the Midwest. She was also not as wealthy as some of the other Ricers.

We met after lunch at the Rice House for the interview. The setting was the dilapidated front porch, and our audience consisted of fellow Ricers. At this point, most of the other Ricers knew of my project and were curious about it. No one left the front porch during the interview. Everyone but me lit up a cigarette as Cindy began.

Cindy Sitco

"I had known about the Rice Diet forever and had planned my escape to Durham for around a decade, but I didn't really believe that I would do it. Everyone said I wouldn't. They'd say, 'Yeah, yeah, the Rice Diet sounds like a good idea, but isn't it a bit extreme?' 'You'll die if you eat only rice and fruit.' 'Besides, how can you afford to go to Durham for a year?'

"When I decided to come to Durham, that was it. I put my business up for sale, gave up my apartment. I sold everything I had. All I kept was my car because I would need that to drive to North Carolina. I felt so free and happy and light. I lost about seven to ten pounds just preparing to come to the Rice House. I didn't tell anybody where I was going, not even my best friend. I did tell my parents, but I made them swear they wouldn't tell anyone. I didn't want any naysayers or even any congratulations. I wanted to be left alone. This was my decision, my life, and I was finally going to live it without interruption. It was such a great feeling to know that at last I was going to focus on me and my weight and be successful at weight loss.

"My parents told some of their friends, and the word got out that I was going to Durham. Everybody was very positive. They threw me a big party at work, and there was a ton of food. Here I am going to Durham because I am too fat to diet at home, and what do people do to mark the occasion? They feed me.

"I had money for about six months on the Rice Diet, and that wasn't nearly enough to pay for all the time I needed to lose my weight and get to goal. My parents gave me the rest of the money. They took it out of their retirement. This surprised me because I thought they were in denial about my weight. When I left Missouri, it was cold and raining. I drove in rain probably until Tennessee. When I arrived in Durham, the sun was shining. I took it as a sign that this was the place for me.

"My last meal before the Rice Diet was in Chapel Hill. I was already in a hotel in Durham, but I drove to Chapel Hill for my Last Supper. I ate a burrito platter at El Rodeo, a Mexican restaurant. I made them make everything extra salty and spicy. I had a margarita the size of a fishbowl. It was not the best meal I ever had, but it was the most satisfying because I knew it would be the last meal for the old me. It was my farewell dinner to myself."

Other Ricers nodded their heads in approval of Cindy's Last Supper. Mexican food is the fantasy of many a dieter. I used to dream of my favorite Mexican food meal while I was on the Rice Diet: a taco and tequito platter from a Tex-Mex restaurant—Anita's—in northern Virginia where I used to live. I announced this to the crowd, and John Griffith, a fellow Ricer sitting on the front porch, seconded my declaration. He too was a fan of Anita's and said he had the T-shirt to prove it.

I was first introduced to John by Abby Felcher. John and Abby were exercise buddies and would walk the Wall together after meals at the Rice House. John was in his late forties and said that he was at the Rice House for health reasons. He wanted to make sure that I depicted him as a person who was dieting for health, not for appearance. However, he was very self-conscious about his looks and wore a long coat throughout the interview. Another Ricer once told me that people do this because they believe a coat will hide the fat. I myself favor long coats.

I met John at the Ninth Street Bakery one afternoon for his interview. We drank Red Zinger tea, which he paid for. John, as promised, wore his Anita's T-shirt. We both sighed and regretted that we would never be able to eat there again. John stirred two packets of artificial sweetener into his tea as he began.

John Griffith

"The first time I came to Durham I had no choice. I was dying. I had hypertension that nobody could control with drugs. I was about seventy-five to one hundred pounds overweight. I didn't think of myself as fat. I didn't even think of myself as angry. That realization came later. My doctor told me that I had a choice—I could go to Durham or die. So what did I do? Nothing. I kept working. I knew I would do it until I dropped. They would find me dead at my desk. All I did was work, and I really loved it. Work was killing me—work and food, but I didn't care because I loved them both. Work was number one because if I didn't work I couldn't buy food. The food was second because it was my secret vice—except it wasn't so secret, because the whole world could see where my attention was.

"I was so fat I was a walking advertisement for food. The thing was, I still went to the gym. Exercised all the time, and it didn't do any good. It was not relaxing because I saw the same people I work with; I would even meet my clients at the gym. I couldn't get away from work. Also, the more I exercised the more I ate because I thought I deserved to eat more! Every night I had my Last Supper and every morning when I promised myself that this would be the day I would begin to lose weight, I would fall off the wagon and then have another Last Supper. I was like a hamster on a treadmill. I couldn't stop. Finally, I made the decision to come to Durham. I just took a leave of absence. Told them I was going on vacation. I didn't say I was going to Durham to diet because I didn't want my competitors to know I was ill. I didn't want my friends or associates to know either. People can smell weakness. I didn't want to let go, but I had to.

"My wife at the time came with me to Durham and helped me get set up in an apartment. It was sort of nice driving here because it was the first time we had been alone in ages. It was like a second honeymoon. I think the drive to Durham was the longest uninterrupted time I ever spent with my wife. It was really sweet. We stopped at all of these tourist places. Spent two days in New York City just walking around and enjoying the sites. Took the ferry around Manhattan. Saw a Broadway show. Ate at some fine restaurants, that sort of thing. Drove on to D.C. and went up to the top of the Washington Monument. Went to the Kennedy Center. Took one of those dinner and dance moonlight cruises on the Potomac. The funny thing was, the closer I got to Durham, the more food was beginning to lose its meaning. For most of my life, food was like this huge gorilla on my back. In Durham all of that left me and I just felt satisfied. Imagine, a man my size living off rice and fruit. My last meal was a meatball sub and four Coors Lights."

So that was how he'd heard of Anita's: he'd passed through northern Virginia on his way to Durham. We promised each other that if we both got to goal weight, we would drive to Anita's for a Mexican foodfest, just once, for old times' sake. That night, I pulled my faded Anita's T-shirt out of the bottom of one of the old boxes that I used as a temporary chest of drawers and slept in it. When I bought that thing, three years before my arrival in Durham, it was so tight I was embarrassed to wear it in public. I keep it as a memento rather than as a piece of clothing. That night I put it on, and it hung off my shoulders and drooped to my knees. That did it. I vowed not to meet John or anyone else at Anita's. Mexican food would never touch my lips again. I was going to get to goal.

Paul Rennard was a friend of John's; they had met at the Rice House. Through John, I got my interview with Paul. Our preliminary meeting took place at the Rice House with John present. The second meeting was with Paul only. We met at Spanky's, a restaurant in Chapel Hill.

I was nervous interviewing Paul. I didn't know him, but had seen him at the Rice House a couple of times. I was apprehensive about getting into a car with some guy I hardly knew. I suggested that I meet him at the restaurant, but he insisted that we go in his car. I reluctantly agreed. He said nothing to me on the ride to the restaurant. He didn't even turn on the radio during the drive. However, once we got inside the restaurant he began to talk up a storm. My fears were unfounded, and I began to relax once we were in Spanky's and Paul opened up.

Paul ordered broiled salmon prepared without salt, butter, or seasoning of any kind. I ordered the same. When his dinner came, Paul cut it into thirds and asked the curious waiter for a carry-out container. He placed two-thirds of his meal in the box and ate the remaining salmon on his plate very quickly. I asked him to explain his behavior, but he refused. I assumed it was his way of eating a little bit of what he wanted without gaining too much weight. I was very conscious of my portion of salmon and cut it in two. I ate half of it and left the other half on my plate. After dinner, the waiter brought a couple of black coffees, and the interview began.

Paul Rennard

"After I had made the decision to come to Durham, or rather my doctors decided I should come here, I fought it all the way. How could I just take off and go to Durham for an unspecified amount of time? What would happen to my business? How could I support my family? All of these worries were running around my head, yet I just didn't see how I couldn't do it. It's not like I had to go to my boss and ask for a leave of absence. I am the boss. Finally, I just had to face up to the fact that Durham was the answer.

"Once I made the decision, everything fell into place, like it was written in the Book of Days or something. It was as though I knew in my soul that I was doing the right thing, I was on the true path. I told my business partners first, and they were very, very supportive. Then I told my family, and they were delighted. I told them right at the dinner table. My youngest boy started to cry. I thought he was sad because I would be going away, but he said he was crying because he was so happy. You see, he had heard me telling my wife that I was so fat I was going to die. Every time he saw me eat he would get scared because he thought I would literally explode. He lived in terror that his dad would die on him. When I told him I was going to lose weight and get healthy, he cried and cried. He asked me if I got thin enough, whether I'd be able to play ball with him. Now it was my turn to cry. I was so fat that I had not been able to play any kind of sports with my kids. Can you believe that? I missed so much in life. That's the hardest part about losing weight. You realize how much was lost because of the fat, and those lost chances can never be returned. It is the feeling of regret that gets you.

"The obstacles I was fearful of never appeared. The only thing that held me back was me, and now I am here on the Rice Diet and I am at peace. My Last Supper before the Rice Diet was a bucket of Kentucky Fried Chicken, a quart of mashed potatoes, and one of those little bowls of gloppy gravy. I had a six-pack of beer with it."

Paul paid for the meal and we walked out of the restaurant and decided to take a stroll down Franklin Street, Chapel Hill's main drag. The evening was warm, and one of the flower ladies was still out with all her wares. I bought a small bouquet and followed Paul to his car. On the drive back to Durham, Paul played the radio and rolled down the window. I leaned back in the deep leather seat and breathed in the smell of heat, car exhaust, and honeysuckle. I turned and saw Paul's profile. For some reason, I still remember his pose. I left the flowers in his car.

I met Timothy Adams through Sylvia Goldman. Timothy was the pet of the older female repeat dieters at the Rice House. He was young, single, cute, and funny, and he would tag along with them on their numerous errands. He was the token son or grandson of the ladies of the dieting community. Timothy had been on several different diet programs and still attended most of them. He would pick and choose from different diets to get the exact match for his diet and exercise preferences. He ate at the Rice House because the Rice Diet had a history to it and that appealed to him. He liked the tradition of it. He also lost weight fast on it. He exercised at the Center for Living because he liked the facilities and the exercise instructors better than those of any other program in Durham. On occasion, Timothy would meet and hang out with dieters on other programs such as Structure House and the Duke Diet and Fitness Center. He especially liked DFC because it was close to his apartment, and he could stop by on his way home to see if there were any good parties happening that evening.

I liked Timothy because he was fun to be around, but he was difficult to interview. It was hard to get a straight answer out of him because he hid his thoughts and feelings behind jokes and wisecracks.

I met with Timothy at his apartment. I had none of the apprehension that I'd had about being alone with Paul; Timothy was a pussycat, a big teddy bear, and a decade younger than I. I didn't see him as a man, but as a boy. Timothy was playful and funny, where Paul was serious and reserved. Tim's apartment was furnished with a plaid couch, crates for end tables, and piles of books, magazines, computer equipment, and sealed boxes.

Timothy brought out orange diet soda and a small bag of rice crackers. He lit a cigar, coughed a little, and opened the sliding glass door so we wouldn't gag on the smoke. He sat very close to me on the couch and leaned back. I giggled, and he moved a little farther away as he became serious and started talking about his Last Supper.

Timothy Adams

"I have all sorts of pre-Rice Diet rituals I do now. My Last Suppers consist of a variety of favorite foods that must be prepared in precise ways. Also, I have this big deal about food pairings, or balances as I call them. The potato chips must be balanced by a highly carbonated Coke in a sixteen-ounce bottle—not a Pepsi, not Coke in a can, not twelve ounces, but sixteen. I want my Last Supper to be as perfect as possible.

"The first time before I went to the Rice House, my mom fixed me her fantastic pot roast with brown gravy and mashed potatoes. That has become my pre-Rice Diet favorite meal. She simmers the roast in Coke for about two hours until it is so tender. Then she makes this really rich brown gravy that is almost black. She makes up these fluffy white potatoes. Heaven. I just reveled in the whole meal because I knew I wouldn't have it again for months and months.

"My sweetest memory is sneaking out of my house with my hidden allowance money. I must have been about eight years old. I got on my bicycle and rode to the supermarket. It was the first time I had crossed the highway by myself. I felt like I was on some kind of military mission. I got to the store and bought an Entenmann's pound cake. Not the fat-free kind, but the real thing. The all-butter loaf with ten grams of fat and 220 calories per slice. The sodium is around 290 milligrams per slice. I got home, went up to my room and locked the door and ate the whole thing. I didn't eat it all at once, but rather piece by buttery piece. Took me around three days to eat it. Now, my secret Last Supper is an Entenmann's pound cake. Nobody knows about it but me. It is my ritual, my goodbye. I used to bring the cake with me in my duffel bag, but since I live here now, I just buy one at the store. I know that may sound like I am technically cheating in Durham, but it doesn't actually count because it is before the Rice Diet. Once I start the Diet, I don't cheat."

After the interview, Timothy asked me to drive him to a friend's apartment near Chapel Hill. I couldn't figure out why he didn't want to take his own car, or how he would get home. It was out of my way, but I agreed to do it. En route to his friend's apartment, Timothy had me stop at a video store, a drugstore, and a liquor store. I guess he was planning a private party. I dropped him off at an apartment complex, and he didn't even thank me as he lumbered off into the night with his purchases. I suppose he figured the interview was thanks enough.

I knew Sadie Rosen long before I ever asked her for an interview. I saw her around Durham: at the Ninth Street Bakery, the movies, and of course, the Rice House. She was friendly but always alone. I asked a couple of dieters about her and was told that Sadie was the owner of a multimedia conglomerate. She was from Louisiana and had been coming to the Rice House since 1968. She was married and had children, grandchildren, and even two great-grandchildren. When I asked for an interview, she turned me down, but later phoned me and arranged to meet at Duke Gardens.

I thought it was very strange that anyone would want to meet outside at Duke Gardens in January. I assumed that Sadie was an dotty old eccentric who was used to being indulged because she was rich. Still, I did meet her there, and she explained to me that the gardens were her special place to walk and she did so every day she was on the Rice Diet, no matter what the weather was like. She loved gardening and knew the Latin names of every tree and shrub we passed. As we strolled along the pathways, I switched on my tape recorder, and Sadie picked up her pace almost to a jog. I hurried to catch up with her. She was old and overweight, but fast. She didn't look at me as she started her story.

Sadie Rosen

"When I came to Durham so many years ago, I didn't know how strict the Diet was going to be, so I didn't go on a farewell binge in New Orleans. I figured that I would miss the Cajun food and the breads, but I thought I would be able to have meat, chicken, and fish on the Rice Diet. It wasn't like I was going to live without any food. My friends and family did have a big party for me. I thought I was going to die without my family. They are so dear to me. I am the big fat mama of the whole clan and it was so hard to leave them.

"There were all of these people crying and hugging on me. There were buckets of shrimp, corn, and the usual picnic food for Louisiana. I ate a ton of food at the party, but I always ate a ton of food so it was no big deal for me. Everyone kept kidding me that I would soon be eating rice and fruit on that wacky diet, and I laughed along with them, but I didn't really believe them. I had read about the Rice Diet and knew that it was mainly rice and fruit, but I focused on the *mainly* part and thought surely they would include other foods. My doctor told me that I would be on rice and fruit until all my levels—blood sugar, cholesterol, triglycerides, and blood pressure—were down to the normal range. Still, my mind just wouldn't accept that.

"About three days before I drove up to Durham, I got this rush of euphoria that I was going to change, that my life would no longer be the same stifled, depressed world of a fat lady—you know the type, jolly on the outside and miserable on the inside. I was changing even though I hadn't even lost a pound. I felt myself freeing up inside. I was very, very happy, but in a quiet, satisfied way. At the same time, I was kind of nervous. Maybe they did only serve rice and fruit in Durham. It's called the Rice House for a reason.

"When I first came to Durham, the Rice House was really strict and Kempner was king. He would take away Ricers' money, credit cards, and car keys so they couldn't cheat.

"I began to worry that I would be without my old standbys in

Durham. I wouldn't have a Butterfinger handy when I needed a little reward. I wouldn't have a bag of Ripple potato chips around for when I got really angry. I wouldn't have a hunk of cheddar cheese and two bottles of Guinness Stout to soothe away the pain of just plain living.

"Before I left New Orleans, I bought my favorite secret food passions and hid them in a box of clothing. I shipped the clothing UPS to the Holiday Inn in Durham. That way, my husband would never find the food that I was taking with me.

"My husband drove with me to Durham and then took the car back. He did that so I would have to walk everywhere and I would lose weight through exercise if nothing else. Also, in their letter to prospective dieters, the staff at the Rice House discouraged bringing cars to Durham.

"My husband spent one night with me at the hotel and then left for home. I was supposed to start the Rice Diet that next morning, but I didn't. Instead I spent the next two days wallowing in the food I loved so well. I was thrilled to be in Durham, but I was scared to death. What if I couldn't do it? What if the Rice Diet couldn't cure me? Maybe I was just a total failure. I thought of all these things while pacing and consuming bag after bag of potato chips. I couldn't walk across the floor without crunching down on something. I promised myself that I would begin the Rice Diet the next day.

"I was full from all of that bingeing, but I just couldn't get the idea of one final pizza out of my head. I loved pizza and the greasier the better. I knew if I didn't have one last pizza, I would die. I was standing there in that hotel room in my nightgown and flip-flop sandals and knew I had to have a pizza. I grabbed my raincoat and the one credit card I had smuggled into Durham. I was totally alone in a city I had never been in before, and I had no idea where to find a pizza at nine p.m. on Sunday. I ran out of the hotel and hailed a taxi. I told him to find me a pizza joint and fast. He didn't even blink an eye. I guess he was used to fat ladies in Durham who go on wild goose chases for pizza parlors. He went all over Durham, but couldn't find one open. Finally, he found a place just before it was closing. The proprietor didn't want to unlock the door and let me in because he was going home. I pleaded and begged and slapped my American Express card against the window, and he finally relented. I got this huge pepperoni pizza with extra cheese.

"Okay, mission accomplished, but how was I going to sneak this big red-and-white pizza box through the hotel lobby teeming with Ricers? They would all know that I was cheating, and I hadn't even been in Durham a week. I was so embarrassed. I should have just tossed the whole thing into the trash, but I wanted the pizza more than anything in this world. I turned the box sideways, tucked it under my raincoat and walked as quickly as I could across the lobby. By the time I got to my room the cheese and pepperoni had slid off into one corner of the pizza. I didn't care. I ate the whole thing and even scraped the dried cheese off the box. Every time I come to Durham now, it is the same ritual—one last pizza."

After she finished talking I turned off the tape recorder and asked her if she needed a ride anywhere. It was too cold for a woman her age to be out. She assured me that she was fine and would walk the five miles back to the Rice House. Not to be outdone, I agreed to walk with her. I left my car in the parking lot of Duke Gardens and hiked to the Rice House with Sadie leading. It took me two days to go back and pick up my car. I, like Sadie, had to walk everywhere in Durham. I lost four pounds in those two days and vowed to restrict my driving as much as possible.

I met Elaine Sutton, a history professor from a large university in the Northeast, at breakfast at the Rice House. I sat at her table one morning and asked her what her story was—how did she end up at the Rice House? Elaine looked like she was interested, and I explained to her what I was doing. She too was curious as to why we all ended up in Durham. She found most people at the Rice House to be very successful in their careers, but failures at losing weight and keeping it off.

The Rice House was fairly peaceful when I set up my tape recorder and notebook. Most people were at a cooking class. Elaine didn't like to participate in those classes because the temptation to cheat was too great, and if she ate any food off the Diet, she would unleash her appetite and destroy all of her good work. I knew exactly what she meant. I attended one of those cooking classes: the food, while low in calories, fat, and sodium, was laid out in such a beautiful fashion that it awakened my love of eating. After that class I went out and cheated a little on the Diet and gained two pounds.

Elaine and I sat across from each other on the overstuffed couches in the Rice House living room. I sank deep into the couch and struggled to keep my tape recorder from rolling off my knees. Elaine sat very straight on the edge of her seat. On her lap was her book bag. From it, she pulled out a tiny tape recorder and popped in a cassette. She was taping the interview also. She said she wanted it for her personal files. I glanced up at my name on the Century Board (the board at the Rice house that displays the names of recent dieters who have lost one hundred pounds or more) and Elaine nodded her approval. She began.

Elaine Sutton

"Coming to Durham was the profound turning point of my life. After I answered the Call, everything just opened up for me. I took a leave of absence from my job; I have tenure so I can do that sort of thing. I told my colleagues that they would have to carry on without me for six months to a year. I resigned from all committees and stopped my research. Everyone was a bit peeved by my behavior, but I didn't care. The funny thing was that I used to really care what people thought of me. After I made the decision to come to Durham, I didn't give a tinker's damn one way or another about anything but getting to Durham and losing my weight.

"My husband was put out by all of it. At first he was very supportive, but then reality set in and he got a little defensive. My sons, on the other hand, were all for it. They were tired of having a fat mother.

"The department had one of those typical potlucks for me. You know, the kind where everyone brings a casserole of something vegetable-like and organic with a gob of cheese on top. Add to the mix an assortment of pies and cakes and a few bottles of domestic wine. It was the first potluck I ever attended where I didn't bring a dish. Usually, I brought several dishes, and I would stand back proudly as people oohed and ahhed over the food I prepared. This time I didn't care. I really enjoyed the potluck and ate what I wanted and as much as I wanted. I ate two or three desserts. What did I care? I was going to go to Durham and lose all the weight anyhow. What did three or four more pounds mean?

"I didn't tell anyone I was on the Rice Diet. My colleagues just assumed I had cancer or something and was going for treatment. My husband and children knew the truth, but nobody else. Why tell anyone anyway? They would just try to discourage me.

"I drove to Durham by myself. I detoured to this little country inn near Middleburg, Virginia, and had my Last Supper. I had a Ploughman's Lunch, which consisted of homemade white bread cut very thick and slathered with sweet butter, a hunk of good cheese—in my case a Stilton—and a ripe tomato slice. I had a mug of sparkling apple cider with it. I felt so peaceful inside with such a simple satisfying meal. I just couldn't understand why I was cursed with obesity and couldn't enjoy food like that whenever I was hungry. Still, I accepted the fact that I could not. Now, when I return to the Rice House I have my Ploughman's Lunch, but this time I have the French version made with paté."

She clicked off her tape recorder, pulled out a piece of paper from her book bag, scribbled what I assumed was her name and number on it and handed it to me. The interview was over. We walked out of the Rice House together and got into our cars. Days later when I was cleaning out my purse, I found Elaine's note. It was not her address but an instruction, a quotation from Winston Churchill admonishing, "Never, never, never give up." I still carry it in my wallet as a reminder and a talisman.

Abby Felcher used her Journey experience as a chance to meet up with fellow pilgrims on the road to Durham. I revealed Abby's Call experience in chapter 3, and I often refer to her interview because she left an impression on me. Abby took such joy in living and found something unique and wonderful about everyone she met. She told me that she was not going to be one of those old ladies who join the "ain't it awful club." To her, each day was always better than the day before, and she was improving in every way. Abby warned me to watch out for those in the "ain't it awful club" because they were always scouting for new members. I promised her that I would never look back on the past with longing.

It seemed like Abby knew everyone in Durham, and after she agreed to be interviewed, she told her friends what a kick she got out of it. People called me up and asked when they would get their turn to tell their story.

Abby Felcher

"Every time I go to the Rice House, I eat all the way down I-95 on the way back to Durham—stuff I would never eat anyplace else. I start with dining out at a lot of really good restaurants before I pack to go to Durham. Middle Eastern food is a favorite, and I search for the best hummus before I leave. Sometimes I go to the Homestead or White Springs [resorts]. They have incredible food. At home, believe it or not, I am in a Gourmet Dining Club. We go out once a month to some great restaurant. I never eat a lot when I am out with friends because you are not really supposed to pig out at these places. Instead, you are supposed to enjoy the presentation of the food. You marvel at the saltiness of the prosciutto as it contrasts with the perfect sweetness of the ripe melon. You comment on the delicately constructed dessert that is about a foot high and two inches wide—that sort of thing. At those functions I taste a bit of this and that and pay a ton of money for it, then go home and have some microwave popcorn and a Dr Pepper.

"The wonderful part about going to Durham is that I get to eat to my heart's content and to my heart's detriment in South Hill, Virginia. I get those good southern sausage biscuits and make sure the sausage has extra sage. I eat fried chicken and mashed potatoes with butter and gravy and fried pies for dessert. I drink gallons of sweet tea. I do it all with no regrets. The very first time I went to Durham I ate a whole Meat Lovers pizza at Pizza Hut and enjoyed every single bite. I can honestly say it was the first time I ate without feeling guilty. It was so good. I will never forget it.

"I have met up with several others who drive down 95 on the way to the Rice House and consider South Hill the Last Supper stop. It is like old home week. We all get together and eat and eat and swap stories before we enter Durham County and before we start the Rice Diet. Once in Durham, I never, never cheat, but before I get there—anything goes."

After the interview, Abby took me on a tour of Durham and pointed out things I had never noticed before, such as stones in an old bridge, the detailed ironwork on forgotten gateways, and house after house leaning on uneven wooden frames. Abby had an interest in everything and looked and acted decades younger than her peers. We started to go places together, and she was right at home at an elegant dinner party or a frat-house mixer.

A year later, when I received the news that Abby was dying, I drove to her home and spent a few hours with her. Abby was busy planning a motorcycle trip through California with a much younger male friend. She wanted to die as she had lived—loving life and riding down the highway on a motorcycle with the full sun in her ageless eyes.

Unlike the people I interviewed, I did not have a formal Last Supper. I figured I had already had too many Last Suppers in my life, and that was why I ended up in Durham. My actual Last Supper was a bowl of plain white rice from one of the Duke University Medical Center's many cafeterias. I sat alone at the aluminum table and ate my bowl of rice as slowly as I could, mindful of every bite. The simple act of eating rice was full of meaning. I wanted that memory to be anchored in me so I could recapture it when I needed a reminder of why I was in Durham and how I got there.

I found that the people I interviewed had similar Journey experiences. Their story was my story. Like Judy Moscovitz, I sold everything to come to Durham, except for the twelve-year-old Toyota Tercel which I drove cross-country to the Rice House. Like all of us, I believed that the Journey was a fabulous period of expectation and joy. We were on the way to the diet capital of the world, where miracles would be found, cures would be obtained, and a lifetime of thinness available to all who were willing to spend the time and money to attain it. That belief and the commitment that supports it pours money into the Durham economy and keeps it thriving.

Last Supper Restaurant

We who are about to diet choose our last supper selections from this menu of our favorite fat- salt- and sugar-laden foods. Our selections may be accompanied by French or Italian bread.

Appetizers

Goldfish crackers

Potato chips, Cheetos, and Chili Cheese Fritos

Main Courses

Pizza, all kinds

Mexican food, especially chimichangas

Chinese spare ribs and fried wontons

Foot-long meatball and cheese sub

Kentucky Fried Chicken Extra Crispy

Chicken Cordon Bleu

Lasagna

Pot roast

Side Dishes

Thick-cut French fries with the skins on

Mashed potatoes with cream gravy

Macaroni and cheese (homemade or by Stouffer's)

Beverages

Alcohol—all kinds

Starbucks double mocha coffee breve
(made with half-and-half)

Sixteen-ounce bottles of Coca-Cola, chilled with no ice

Desserts

Pound cake

Cookie dough ice cream

A box of See's candies

A box of mints from Marshall Field's

five Durham: Living Off the Fat of the Land

During the first twenty years of its existence, the Rice Diet generated twenty-eight million dollars. We dieters account for over one hundred million dollars of the Durham economy's revenue. We spend money on the diet programs, buy clothes, go to movies, buy cars, rent accommodations, and even buy houses. Owning a house or apartment in Durham is a good investment, because all of us know that sooner or later we will end up back in Durham on a diet program.

All sorts of Durham businesses cater to us. The business owners and advertisers realize what an opportunity incoming dieters represent. Theater seats in Durham are larger than they are elsewhere to accommodate our girth. Theater managers know that dieters are new in town and have nothing much to do except go to the movies a lot. Durham caters to us by providing plus-size clothing shops, alteration and tailoring establishments, cooking schools that specialize in low-fat meal planning, restaurants that serve Ricer-type meals, and singles mixers that are for large-sized clients only.

Some businesses cater to us in a negative way. As one anonymous Ricer puts it, "Oh, I'll tell you something crazy about this town. I never saw anything like it. Everywhere you go, I mean everywhere, they got these sandwiches for sale. I went into a tailor's shop the other day, and there was a pile of those sandwiches on a counter. You can wolf down a couple while you're waiting for your dry cleaning, for Christ's sake."[20] Durham is full of restaurants featuring all-you-can-eat buffets. Many gourmet food shops lure starving dieters in with trays filled with free bite-size delectables. Ice cream stores provide free samples of any flavor to interested customers, and the food courts at local malls hawk their wares by handing out food to all passersby.

Our impact is not felt just in the economic sector, but in the local emerging arts community as well. We patronize the arts because we come from large cities that have diversified cultural outlets. We also have time on our hands while in Durham and are able to volunteer, join theater groups, and actively participate in local productions.

Businesses that are not listed in the Chamber of Commerce publications profit from the diet population as well. Prostitutes (or commercial sex workers, as they like to be called) cater to incoming dieters and can often be found in the public areas of local hotels at happy hour. Some have an exclusive and very secret clientele and can only be located after strict precautions have been observed. I met a young man who catered to the sexual appetites of female dieters and made three hundred dollars an hour for his expertise. He was once rewarded with a brand-new silver Porsche by a satisfied customer.

We have benefited Durham's financially strapped widows also. Many are left with big houses and small incomes. Renting to Ricers on a weekly basis helps fill the void in their lives and in their bank accounts, and some have been doing it for forty years or more. We get a list of rooms for rent from the Rice Diet office. These rooms can be elaborate or spartan. Most rentals consist of standard bedrooms furnished with a double bed, a worn dresser, a table, a nightstand, a phone, and a television. The bathroom is often down the hall and must be shared with other dieters who may be on different programs. The weekly rates include laundry and linen service, but no kitchen privileges. We are there to diet, not to dine.

Some people come to Durham to diet and leave. They are tourists who just want to get thin, leave, and come back for tune-ups as needed. For others, Durham is much more. It is the home they have been searching for all their lives—even if they weren't aware that they were looking for one.

Irene Groves feels that way about Durham. It is the only place where she truly comes alive. I talked to Irene as I drove her to one of her medical appointments at Duke. Later we had a more formal interview on the porch of the Rice House. Irene smoked one cigarette after another as she talked. She knew that her doctors wanted her to give up her habit, but she believed she was too old to stop now.

It was difficult for me to keep from choking from all that smoke, but Irene was oblivious to my discomfort. Between puffs she informed me that she considered herself a very youthful and active senior citizen.

Other Ricers had finished their meals and were congregating on the porch. Every time anyone attempted to sit in a chair near us, Irene stared him or her down, and the person would move on to another seat. Irene didn't want too many people hearing her story because she felt it was none of their business. She didn't mind telling me or having her interview recorded because she considered that "scientific and historical." She leaned over and spoke carefully into my tape recorder.

Irene Groves

"I will never forget my first summer in Durham. It was just like going to summer camp when I was a child, except it was summer camp for adults and fat ones at that. In Durham, I was alone for the first time since I was a child. I went straight from my parents' home to my husband's. We had a pretty good life, but when he died I decided to come to Durham. I had known about Durham all my life, but just never got around to coming here.

"I'd been fat off and on throughout my life. I was actually a very skinny kid. My mother used to give me Eagle Brand sweetened condensed milk to put weight on me. It didn't work. I remained skinny until I was around thirty-two years old. Then I gained about twenty-five pounds in a year. I was married and working hard and just didn't have time to address my weight problem. I joined Weight Watchers, of course, but couldn't stick to it, and I hated going to those meetings. They were on Thursday nights at seven p.m. I will never forget the effort it was to go to them. I would rush out from work, get on the freeway, get stuck in traffic, get to the meeting late, and my weight would be up three pounds and that would make me so nervous. Then some thin lady would give us a lecture about weighing our food. I hated Weight Watchers. Still, I knew I had to do something about my weight, but I didn't know when. It was always: After the fall shipments come in, I will diet. After the children leave home, I will diet. After I pay off the house, I will diet. Oh, I went to TOPS [Take off Pounds Sensibly] too, but never lost more than twenty-eight or thirty pounds. I just couldn't devote any time to my weight. When my husband died, I knew it was time.

"Do you know that I didn't have any female friends? I was too busy working to make friends. In Durham, I had the time to make friends. The first day at the Rice House, I sat at a table full of women and just joined in the conversation. It was wonderful. We went shopping together, to the movies. Got my hair dyed blonde and cut in a little bob instead of a gray bun knotted at the back of my head. I started wearing contact lenses. I bought my first real wardrobe in Durham. Really. I worked every day of my life, but I always wore the same thing—a long black shapeless dress to hide my bulk, thick black stockings, and sensible black shoes. I was totally drab—totally lifeless.

"I met my best friend, Daisy, my first day at the Rice House. We had similar backgrounds. We both owned companies. We had been married to much older men. Both of us had a history of miscarriages. Of course, we were both fat, so we had something in common right there. It was like we recognized something in each other. Having a best friend was the most wonderful thing that ever happened to me, and it wouldn't have happened if I hadn't been on the Rice Diet.

"Coming to Durham and the Rice House changed my life. I started out on the Rice Diet and then went to DFC. DFC is fantastic, and they really cater to dieters. Their focus is education and behavior modification. The time before last, I went to Structure House. Their whole thing is that obesity has a psychological basis and you have to get to the root cause of your overeating. I loved the other programs, but I always return to the Rice Diet. It works for me. The others are fabulous and make you feel great. I learned everything there is to know about calories, fat, and sodium counts. I know what to eat, when to eat, and even why I eat, but for some reason I can't seem to lose all of my weight. I lose some weight, but then begin to put it back on. When I follow the Rice Diet, I lose weight and keep losing it. I guess it's the fact that the Rice Diet had Dr. Kempner. He created the whole diet culture [in Durham]. Without his influence, Durham would be just another hick town.

"I like the Rice Diet because it is always the same. It is so good to know that there is a place to come to in Durham. It is like knowing there is always a room for you at home, left just like it was when you were young. Durham is like that to me. It is my true home. It is where my heart really lives."

I left Irene on the front porch puffing away on another cigarette. Now that the interview was over, some Ricers sat down next to her and lit up their smokes. I walked back to my house wondering if I would still be up to dieting when I was seventy-five. Would I still find the motivation? And what was it that drove Irene to diet? Surely not her health, because the cigarettes alone were capable of killing her. Was it vanity? She never said, and I didn't think to ask her. That night, before I went to bed, I promised myself that if I lived to be seventy-five I would not be dieting. Instead, I would do everything that was bad for my health and all that society forbids. I would eat a load of fat and calories. I would drink to excess. I would smoke continuously, take drugs, and have unprotected sex if I could find the opportunity to do so.

Dorothy McCarthy, like Irene, found her true home in Durham. She came into the Rice House each morning dressed as if she had stepped out of a magazine. Her hair, makeup, and nails were always perfectly done, and her clothes were expensive and pressed. Her jewelry was spare, but impressive. She was also well-armed. She carried a tiny pearl-handled pistol in her Fendi bag and kept a loaded .357 Magnum under the front seat of her car. I never got a look at the Magnum, but she did show me the pistol.

I liked Dorothy right away, and we started to walk together after meals. That is how I got her interview. Dorothy would not sit for more than fifteen minutes at a time. She figured that she would burn more calories standing than sitting and even more if she was walking. Consequently, my talks with Dorothy were on the move.

I met her at Duke Towers for the interview. Her apartment was a jumble of clothes, makeup, magazines, books, framed family photos, and bags of goodies from high-end shops—I. Magnum, Barney's, Neiman Marcus, Marshall Field's, Bloomingdale's, Hermes, Armani Emporium, Fendi, and even Tiffany's. As she searched through piles of stuff to find her pedometer, I asked if she ordered her purchases online or through catalogs: there wasn't a Bloomingdale's for three hundred miles. She informed me that her maid buys the things she needs and sends them to her. Her maid also keeps a detailed record of what Dorothy wears to which function. All of her purchases are logged on a CD-ROM. I was stunned that anyone would live a life that required a CD-ROM of clothing. Before I could find a place to sit, Dorothy had me out of the door and walking briskly around the courtyard at the Towers. As she chugged ahead of me, exaggerating the movement of her hips and widening her gait, she yelled back her story.

Dorothy McCarthy

"My husband brought me to Durham the first time. I have diabetes and went to a doctor in Dallas, and he said that as bad off as I was, the Rice Diet was the only hope for me. I wasn't even very fat at the time, but I was fat enough that it was really bothering my health. My diabetes was not controlled by insulin, and then my heart started to go. I got all sorts of vascular problems, and well, the Rice Diet was the only thing that could help me. That's where all the terminal cases end up, you know, at the Rice House. Dr. Kempner was there at the time, and he did save me. It's the rice that cures you. They haven't even begun to find out what rice can do for you, but Kempner knew.

"My husband stayed with me for a month and got me set up in an apartment. I stayed here [Duke Towers] the first time I came, and it was a revelation to me. I didn't know people could behave that way. At first I was shocked—the language, the attitude, the sex, and the sheer amount of fat people—but I got used to it.

"After my husband left I took up with some women, and we began to walk and exercise together. I started to get some independence and enjoy it. I wrote my first check in Durham—it's true. Can you imagine in this day and age a woman who has never written a check on her own? I didn't have to. My husband took care of all of the finances, and I took care of the house and children, as well as the social obligations of my husband's career. That's how things worked then. In Durham, I didn't have that security. I was on my own, and I loved every minute of it. I was off all my medication within six weeks of treatment at the Rice House. It was as though someone lifted this huge boulder off of my shoulders. I got well and lost eighty-two pounds on the Rice Diet. I went home a healthy, happy, and very thin woman!

"My family didn't know what to say to me. They were not used to seeing me so thin, and I think it frightened them. Also, I was an independent woman now and didn't need them to do for me like I used to. I could do things for myself. I flew out to Durham with my husband and drove home to Texas in a brand-new car. It was a sporty little Mercedes-Benz—silver with blue interior. My husband about flipped, but I didn't care. It was the first thing I actually bought for myself without consulting anyone. I would have never had the guts to do anything like that if I hadn't gone to Durham.

"I live in Texas—at least my body does—but my heart belongs to Durham. I come alive here. I come back to the Rice House regularly because that is the only way I can keep the weight off. No diet compares to the Rice Diet, and the only place you can find that is in Durham."

Dorothy signaled to me that the interview was over. She had to meet with her personal trainer. I was amazed that, after our hike, she was going to continue to exercise. She told me that our walk was just a warm-up, and on a typical day, she exercises for four hours. No wonder she was so thin. I walked to my car, embarrassed that the hike had done me in.

I met Joe Johnson on the stadium steps at Duke. Joe believed that running up and down the steps increased weight loss. He didn't want to stop too long to talk to me because he was anxious to get his exercise routine over for the day. It was impossible for me to interview him while we huffed and puffed and coughed our way up the steps, so I arranged to meet him later in Chapel Hill at an Italian restaurant. He was a gracious and interesting dinner companion and enjoyed telling his story as much as he did eating the meal of plain pasta with salt-free marinara on the side. Joe is the co-owner of a professional sports team and has sent several of his players to the Rice House before spring training.

Joe Johnson

"What does Durham mean to me? Home of the brave and the morbidly obese. It is home to me and a bunch of other fatsos. Really, we all end up in Durham sooner or later. Every lost soul and homeless person shows up in Durham, because it is the last outpost. That's what I consider Durham to be—the city at the end of the world. It is where I really started to live, and it is where I will die. I know that. I even know how I will die—congestive heart failure. That or emphysema. I have that too, you know. Either one will kill me and maybe both. Doesn't matter because I will die in Durham.

"I have been on all of the diet programs here. I started out at Structure House because I read about it in my wife's *Lear* magazine. She had it lying around, and I just flipped through the pages. My eyes fell on this article on Durham and how the fat of the world go there and dump their tonnage and begin life over.

"That's exactly what I needed to do—begin my life over. I called the Structure House and went up over the weekend. I thought I would be there about a week or two, just enough time to get focused on the diet, and then I could go home and follow the diet there. Not a chance in hell of that ever happening. Home is hell because people are always eating. I stayed at Structure House for two months and lost fifty pounds. I felt great. My wife wasn't thrilled, but I was.

"I kept the weight off for about six months, and then it just started to come back. I gained eleven pounds my first weekend home, but leveled off for a while. Then, after six months, I started gaining around ten pounds a month. I was eating low fat—no dairy, no sugar, no alcohol—but that didn't seem to matter.

"The next time I came to Durham was about three years later. By then I weighed about three hundred pounds, maybe more. I went to the Duke Diet and Fitness Center. I stayed there for a while, but the weight loss was too slow. Then I went to the Center for Living, because the focus is on prevention and they really are into preventing heart disease. It was too late for me. They found I had congestive heart failure and that was about it. I couldn't exercise because I had a pain in my chest all the time. Then I found out I had emphysema. I thought I couldn't breathe because I was so fat. Finally, out of desperation, the doctors at CFL sent me to the Rice House and to Dr. Kempner. I lost two hundred and fifty pounds on the Rice Diet in a year and a half. I have kept it off for over a decade now. I come back to Durham all the time. It is the only way I can stay alive."

Joe's story was a moving one and it brought tears to my eyes. I was amazed that someone could lose so much weight in a relatively short time. Joe walked me to my car. I hugged him and wished him well. He smiled and waved as I drove off. I was sure that he was going back to the stadium to run the steps. He was a dedicated man.

When I started collecting dieting tales, I had put a notice in the newspaper asking for Ricer stories. Paula Mason was one of the first to respond. She is a child psychologist by profession, but makes her living as a writer and an inspirational speaker. She had devoted her life to "helping others find their true paths." She wanted to meet with me and be interviewed because she believed that people should hear about how powerful it is to be able to be in Durham and lose weight.

I met her at a shelter at Eno River State Park. Paula went to the Eno for her daily meditation. She found the peaceful surroundings conducive to relaxation and deep thought. Today, however, the park was crowded with students from a fourth-grade class. They were there to take specimens of the river for a class science project. Paula resented the presence of the children. It was clear she didn't like them; perhaps that's why she left her profession. Admittedly, it was hard to hear with all of their noise. Paula and I walked farther back into the park to a more secluded spot. As we slowly and carefully maneuvered our way over the rocks, I felt my fanny pack to make sure I'd brought enough batteries. We found a big rock to sit on and Paula began.

Paula Mason

"Durham's sacred ground to me. It is my soul's home. I know that sounds silly to the uninitiated, but it's true. I have been fat and ill most of my life. Due to my arthritis and my limited mobility I couldn't exercise much, and I just got fatter and fatter. I would have physical therapy and paddle around in the pool, but I lost absolutely no weight. I would feel better after exercise, but I wouldn't be any thinner. I came to the Rice Diet and just stayed. It was the first time I felt truly accepted.

"There was a lot of tension in the air. Don't get me wrong. Fat people are angry people. There is no such thing as a jolly fat man. Look at the Rice House. Everyone there is angry, but it is a righteous sort of anger. We have taken a back seat in life and have been treated like second-class citizens because of weight. It really is an injustice! It makes me so mad when people try to tell me that it isn't. Look at me! I am fat, I am handicapped, and I am a woman. Don't tell me about injustice. I have three strikes against me before I walk into a room.

"The Rice House is truly the only place I feel at home. Everyone is there for the same reason: to lose weight. We all rally and support each other. We don't have to pretend or put on any facade. We are what we are. We accept each other, and we speak to each other in a kind of shorthand. We don't have to explain much because we have similar lives. We are fat people in a world that values thinness. We scare people.

"I was so passive before I came to Durham and so timid. Looking back, I am disgusted by how I let people treat me. Durham is where I found my voice. I went through a personal transformation. As my body got thinner, my soul got stronger, and I just didn't take any crap from anybody. I was bold and spoke up. I went through college and graduate school and never said a word in class. I always agreed with people even though I was seething inside. At the Rice House I started listening to people and learning a few things about the world. I learned to just open up my voice and let the chips fall where they may. I didn't care if I angered people.

"My best friend Polly, whom I met at the Rice House, told me I was a mouse when I started the program and a lion when I left. That's true. When I came to Durham and began the Rice Diet, I didn't know what I wanted to be when I grew up. I didn't know what my purpose was. After two weeks of eating rice and fruit, I decided I wanted to be the Weather Underground of fat people. I wanted to avenge fat people all over the world. I wanted to spray paint over ads that ridiculed fat people. I wanted to save fat kids from shame and degradation. I wanted to free other people like I freed myself.

"In Durham, I could walk down the street in Lycra bike shorts at my fattest, and nobody batted an eye. I went swimming at Duke Towers in a two-piece bathing suit and nobody cared. It was fabulous. I felt sexy and healthy and powerful. That is the beauty of Durham. I feel powerful in Durham."

I remembered my shopping spree with Sylvia Goldman and her friends. They were worried that I didn't know what looked good on me. They were right. I had always settled for what covered and fit rather than what actually flattered my body. We went to a bathing suit outlet near Apex, and I spent hours trying on suits until we found the perfect one—a simple black one-piece with a square neck in a size twelve. A size twelve! How old was I the last time I could fit into a twelve? I couldn't remember. I loved that suit, and when I wore it I felt powerful. I knew what Paula felt.

After the interview, we made our way back to the entrance of the park and said our good-byes. I saw Paula at the Rice House the next day and sat at her table. She ruled the table like a fierce hostess. She made sure that everyone was included in the conversation, and all were entertained by her wit and educated by her insight. To this day, when I return to the Rice House, I can find Paula at one of the tables, happy to be there.

Kendra Shaw also believes that Durham is her true home. A thirty-five-year-old accountant, Kendra left her husband behind in Cleveland, perhaps for good. I had seen Kendra around Durham with groups of dieters. She was always one of the first in the Rice House each morning. I couldn't keep my eyes off her. She was very beautiful, like a young, oversized Elizabeth Taylor. She was quite fat but very tall, and she had a queenly way about her and a low, breathy voice. She was aware of her effect on people and delighted in it. Although she was married, she would often date fellow Ricers and was known to have broken a heart or two.

We met at the Rice House right after breakfast. Kendra was there before me, ready to give her story. She was decked out in a red tunic with matching leggings. I didn't know you could buy leggings that size, even in Durham. The red set off her dark complexion and long black hair. She squeezed my hand and winked as I turned on the tape recorder. I just shook my head, smiled at her, and sighed. Her current boyfriend came over, sat down next to her, and put his arm territorially around her broad shoulders and she began.

Kendra Shaw

"I love Durham, simply love it. I've never had so much fun in my life as I have in Durham. It is like going back to college. When I first got here, I went on Duke Diet and Fitness Center, and it was one party after another. I lost forty pounds in six months and really started to look good. I had to go home for a while because my husband was getting upset that I was having such a good time in Durham. He just didn't get it. Dieting is supposed to be hard and painful, but I was having this fabulous time. I think he was jealous that I had any free time. I went to the movies with groups of people, then went for coffee afterwards. I played volleyball every weekend with people from all of the other diet programs. It was great.

"In Durham, we are surrounded by people just like us and we have the time to devote to diet and exercise. Weight loss takes a lot of time and effort. Thin people don't understand that, and fat people know it but don't want to accept it. To maintain my weight loss I had to exercise at least two hours a day, walk seven miles, and eat twelve hundred calories or less a day. Right there, that shoots the whole day. When I got home, I kept the weight off for a few months, but then it gradually just came back on. I was so lonely.

"The second time I came to Durham I went on the Rice Diet. It wasn't as glamorous as the other programs, but it sure worked. I lost forty pounds my first month on program. I went on to lose a hundred pounds. I gained most of it back, but I am here and taking it off again.

"The great thing about Durham and the Rice Diet is that it never changes. I hate change, it unnerves me. Most fat people feel that way. Durham looks the same to me year after year, and even though Kempner is dead I can still hear his voice in my ear asking, 'Did you lose?' There is something so comforting about that, something I don't get anyplace else but Durham."

I knew what she meant. When I left the Rice House I was afraid to go back, afraid that all would be different from the way I had remembered it. When I finally did return after being gone for a year, it was as though I had never left. No one was surprised to see me. Even my name tag was untouched.

Because Durham becomes some people's true home, it also becomes a hindrance to weight loss. It is easier to be fat in Durham than anywhere else because you are not in the minority. The city is full of other fat people on diet programs, and the community is used to seeing really obese people. To some Ricers, this ease of living makes dieting harder.

Richard Stokes is one of those who found Durham an easy place to be accepted. He is the owner of a chain of fast-food restaurants. Richard made a living selling high-fat, high-calorie, mass-marketed food to the public for years and became a victim of his own success.

I interviewed Richard at the pool at Duke Towers, even though the pool was drained and it was the dead of winter. The day was cold even for February but very sunny. Richard wore a lightweight jogging suit. He believed that a fat person should not wear a coat in the winter or use air conditioning in the summer because these actions interfered with one's metabolism. Also, he reasoned, he would lose more weight if his body had to fight to maintain a temperature of 98.6 degrees. Consequently, he shivered through the winter and sweated all summer.

Returning Ricers just back in town would stop to chat with Richard. It was as though they wanted to check in with him and pay their respects. He was well-known in the community and had been around for a long time. Even those who didn't know Richard personally knew who he was.

Richard was lying in one of the lounge chairs near the empty pool, holding one of those reflective shields up to his already heavily lined face. I guess he wanted even more sun damage. I had never seen one of those contraptions except in the movies, and it made me laugh that Richard could act so affected. I took off my parka and pulled off my gloves. If he could stand the cold, then so could I. I turned on the tape recorder and huddled close to Richard. I was hoping that between our enlarged body masses we would be able to generate some serious heat.

Richard Stokes

"I came to Durham for the same reason every other fat person does: for Dr. Kempner and his Rice Diet. The first time I saw the place, I was so disappointed. Durham is really an ugly little town, and the Rice House looked like a dump. I got out of my car and thought, 'So this is the world-famous Rice Diet?' The front porch was rotted and there were a bunch of rickety old rocking chairs and an aluminum glider that looked like they would collapse any minute. Of course there were all these fat people jammed into them. I don't know how the porch or the furniture withstood the weight! I thought there must be some kind of mistake. This could not be the famous Rice House. It looked even worse on the inside. The carpet was completely worn out, there were old cots lined up against the wall, and tiny little chairs clustered in the dining room.

I thought this could not be the Rice House I had been hearing about for years. Then this little dried-up old man sitting in the middle of an old couch pointed his finger at me and asked, 'Did you lose?' That was the famous Dr. Kempner. At first I thought the whole place was full of crazies. It took me a couple of weeks to make the mental adjustment to the Rice House and about that long to find my place in Durham.

"I love Durham, even though it's not much to look at, because it's where I belong. I have been fat off and on most of my life, and I knew that I would end up in Durham someday. At seventy years of age I finally did. I lost 152 pounds on the Rice Diet in nine months. I had a tummy tuck because my apron hung down to my knees and I couldn't even find my dick. After the weight loss and the plastic surgery, I was a new man. I went around the world. I divested myself of most of my businesses. I got married and divorced. I got married again. I looked and felt great, but I found out that I could only look and feel great because of Durham. I felt out of place everywhere else because I felt like I was passing for a thin person when I was really a fat person. I looked thin, but inside I was fat. Thin people just don't get that, but fat people do. That is why I moved to Durham. I feel comfortable here.

"That may be a bad thing now. I am spiraling. I go from one diet program to another, but I never manage to get to goal weight. I hang around with a bunch of other diet dropouts, which doesn't help. Still, it could be worse. I could have gained all of my weight back instead of just half of it."

Richard's story scared me to the core. I couldn't imagine gaining back half my weight. That would be tragic. I would have to be especially vigilant in my efforts to lose weight. Durham was getting comfortable to me. I didn't say any of this out loud, but Richard read my mind and nodded. I thanked him for his interview, grabbed my things, and hurried back to my car. I wanted out of the cold and away from his tale of dieting failure. I didn't want it to rub off on me.

Cynthia Owens also found Durham to be an obstacle to weight loss. Like Richard, she had come to Durham to confront her obesity, lose the weight, and return home. It was easy to live in Durham surrounded by fat people. There wasn't the constant pressure to conform to thinness as there was back home. Cynthia was referred to me by my friend, favorite informant, and scout of new interviewees, Abby Felcher.

I interviewed Cynthia in the living room of my home. I made a pot of tea, and Cynthia relaxed a little and settled back in the chair. I was surprised to find out that she had once rented a room in this very house. She had the room across from mine when she first arrived in Durham. I was amazed at this, and she told me that it was no big deal, that she had rented rooms in dozens of houses all over Durham. She put a coaster on the coffee table, put down her mug, and began.

Cynthia Owens

"The problem with this town is that it is just too easy to get stuck. The first time I came here was right out of college, and I did really well. I got within twenty-five pounds of goal weight. I was so dedicated that I wouldn't even have a cup of decaf coffee outside of the Rice House. I had to go home because my family thought I was thin enough. They thought I was cured. Of course, I wasn't. I came back to the Rice House a couple of years later, and I was less into the Diet and more into the party scene. You see, the deal with the Rice House is that there are all of these hangers-on who aren't really on program, but think they are. They show up when the doctors aren't around so they don't have to pay the medical fees, but they still eat at the Rice House. They aren't fooling anyone, and they aren't losing any weight. They eat three or four dinners a week at the Rice House.

"The first time I was in Durham, I stayed away from those people because I thought they were dangerous. They obviously were failures because they were in no way thin. The second time, I thought they were kind of cool. They worked their way around the Diet without actually being on it.

"The third time I came to Durham, I just stayed. I started out at the Rice House, but drifted over to Duke Diet and Fitness Center and then Structure House. None of them did much good because I wasn't really focused. I kept up my exercise at Center for Living, but I didn't follow any diet program.

"There is this whole group of people who are diet rejects. They just hang around Durham because they are still too fat to go home, but they are doing nothing to lose weight. Most of them are thinner than they were when they came to Durham, but that isn't saying much. They don't have real jobs, but dabble in this and that. Many of them are trust-fund babies, so they don't have to work. They party most of the time and sort of rule the diet community. They are like the bad boys in high school. You know the type, the people who are deemed really cool when they are sixteen years old, but seem like losers at thirty-two.

"In Durham you can postpone growing up indefinitely. I am living in suspended animation. I am not thin, but I am not massively obese. I am not on a diet program, but I am part of diet culture. I guess I am waiting for some sort of sign, some kind of direction."

Cynthia spooked me. She recited her story as if by rote, showing very little emotion. She never looked me in the eye or moved throughout the entire interview. I thought that she might be on an antidepressant or some other medication that made her behave this way. She seemed helpless and almost pathetic. She was very aware of her situation and showed great insight and self-awareness, yet was incapable of doing anything about it. Cynthia was younger than I, probably around thirty, and she was already retired. I knew she didn't work or go to school. She wasn't married or close to anyone. It seemed a horrible way to live, with nothing worthwhile to do. When she left, I made several phone calls to people who meant something to me, just to check in and to keep those connections going. That night I slept with all the lights on.

For me, Durham is neither home nor hindrance. I wasn't looking for a home and never really wanted one. I have a restless nature and am always happier going someplace than actually arriving there. I like the journey.

When I was a child growing up in Trenton, Missouri, population five thousand, I would hear the trains of the Rock Island Railroad as they pulled out of town on their way to someplace else.

The train whistle would blow just as I was drifting off to sleep, and I would wish on that train instead of a star, wish to be someplace else. Some afternoons I would walk to the train depot, sit in the waiting room, and watch the passengers come and go. The diet programs of Durham are like that for me. They are way stations for people going someplace else. To me, Durham is not home, but a waiting room for transitionals like me on the road to thinness. It is a place we pass through, where we leave our old selves behind and create new ones.

six

Rites of Passage

After responding to the Call, Journeying to Durham, and consuming the Last Supper, we are ready to enter the Rice House and the innermost circle of diet culture. At Duke University Medical Center, we go through three days of testing with X-rays, cardiograms, blood counts, and even a blood gases test to measure the oxygen content of our fat-saturated blood. A medical photographer takes a "before" photo of each of us. We take home an "after" photo if and when we reach goal weight. When the tests are completed, we receive instructions to show up at the Rice House the next day for the morning ritual and meals. A week after the tests are completed, each one of us receives the "dead letter." This letter states that unless we stick to the Rice Diet and follow it totally and absolutely without question until goal weight is obtained, we will die an early and painful death.

The creed of the Rice Diet is simple food served plainly. For novices, the Rice Diet consists only of rice and fruit. Later on in treatment, vegetables are added. The rice is plain and boiled, without any salt. The fruit is canned or fresh. Each dieter's daily calorie allotment of calories ranges between four hundred and seven hundred a day. A typical breakfast at the Rice House consists of one half of a grapefruit, two-thirds of a cup of oatmeal, and one cup of Sanka—without cream or sugar. Lunch and dinner are identical:

two-thirds of a cup of rice and two servings of fruit. All of us, no matter how large or small or ill, eat rice and fruit until the staff says otherwise. The physical results of the Diet are felt immediately and resemble the early stages of starvation.

Withdrawing food causes the body to feed on carbohydrates stored in the liver. Dr. Kempner referred to this process as "cooking your own bacon." Ricers refer to it as being an "auto-cannibal." The body makes adaptive changes, and as less food is taken in, less energy is expended. The heartbeat slows down, blood pressure drops, internal organs shrink. Dieters experience severe headaches, lethargy, and disorientation. We call this disorientation "Ricerhead," and its onset signals the body's loss of sodium and potassium. Ricerhead is extremely common in beginning dieters.

Ricers use walking as our main exercise and often walk seven, ten, or even fifteen miles a day. One very ambitious group of Dieters walked all the way to Raleigh—twenty-three miles away! We exercise while consuming very little food and no salt whatsoever. Sometimes the levels of sodium and potassium in the body get too low, and a Ricer will pass out. When this happens, the staff adds toast and tomato juice to the Diet. Other side effects include aching muscles, hair loss, changes in menstrual patterns, and vivid dreaming about food. While on the Rice Diet, I would get up at night and look in the wastebaskets to make sure I hadn't really consumed the food I'd dreamed about.

This harrowing period of side effects lasts about ten days, followed immediately by a brief period of a near-euphoria where one feels light, airy and pure in body and spirit. The headaches depart, and clear thought and excess energy occur. Now the body feeds on its own fat and muscle. Weight loss is twenty-five percent fat, twenty-five percent muscle, and fifty percent water. The face thins out, skin sags, and cheeks hollow as bone structure emerges.

Most of us eat rice and fruit for six weeks. After that time, if all body levels such as blood pressure, blood sugar, and cholesterol are normal and the staff allows it, we are allowed to have vegetables. By this point, significant weight loss has occurred.

Under current management the Rice Diet is totally vegetarian, but when I was on it, very lucky Ricers received chicken twice a week. Receiving chicken was the ultimate compliment, meaning that you were being celebrated as a successful Dieter. Getting chicken was a profound moment in a Ricer's life and demonstrated the success of the Dieter to the entire community. It took me almost four months to receive chicken. When I finally did, I knelt in the middle of the floor in the dining room of the Rice House and raised my hands upward in thanksgiving.

A typical day at the Rice House begins with the morning ritual, which consists of getting weighed, having your blood pressure checked, and reviewing the results of the sodium counts. To ensure that we adhered to the strictness of his diet, Dr. Kempner required urine samples twice a week for sodium tests. The staff posted the results of these tests in a public area of the Rice House. Those of us who had kept to the Diet had very low sodium levels. Every day I looked up my sodium counts, and I was delighted when I got one of the red circles that denoted very low sodium levels. The urine samples insured diet compliance. Those unfortunate Ricers who ate outside the Rice House still had to submit urine samples, and their cheating showed up in high sodium counts. Too many high counts could lead to dismissal from the Diet. Since Kempner's death, urine samples are requested periodically, but the results are not publicly revealed, and there are no red circles.

When I was at the Rice House, the morning ritual ended with viewing photographs of a successful Ricer—one who has reached goal weight. I loved this part of the ritual because it showed me that someone could really lose a tremendous amount of weight on the Diet. The before and after photographs were passed around and enhanced the transformational quality of the Rice Diet. Today at the Rice House before and after photographs are not routinely passed around, but can be found in the promotional materials and in the Rice Diet newsletter.

All of us go through the same initiations to become a Ricer. We all have to weigh in each day, provide urine samples as requested, and eat every meal at the Rice House. We all experience the same hunger. These shared experiences are part of the rites of passage of diet culture. We enjoy the unity and fellowship which comes from shared suffering.

Many us of go from anger about our bodies and our lives to acceptance. We are angry at the world because we are angry at ourselves. Why can't we control our weight? What is wrong with us? Why doesn't the world treat us better? Why don't we treat ourselves better? These are questions we ask ourselves over and over. Acceptance comes through weight loss.

Linda Marletti expressed these feelings when I interviewed her over dinner at Squid's, a seafood restaurant in Chapel Hill. Squid's is popular with dieters because the chef will prepare the entrées without any added salt or butter. The waitstaff is used to dealing with Ricers and does not deny any unusual requests. Linda was happy to tell her story and glad that someone had finally asked her how she felt about her weight loss. She was a newspaper columnist and quite familiar with the interview process. I was eager to interview her because I understood from conversations with others that Linda was a very successful dieter and managed to keep her weight off. I was nervous at first, because Linda was fairly well known and very good at her job. I was merely a graduate student and fellow Ricer. People who recognized her kept coming over to our table during the interview, which added to my apprehensiveness.

Linda Marletti

"I thought I was going to die the first two weeks on program. I used to slap a urine bottle label on my shirt in case I passed out on the street. I was so gung ho the first time I was here that I just walked and walked all the time. I walked through some rough neighborhoods and even walked at night because I thought I was invincible. I just didn't think anything bad could happen to me in Durham.

"I remember exactly what I felt the first time I walked into the Rice House. I opened that old Victorian-style door, and it was as though I took a step into my own life. For the first time, I felt that me and my fat were the same person. To someone thin, this concept sounds absurd. That is because thin people don't see their very flesh as alien. Fat people do. I was constantly at war with it, but it never left my side. It was my side! But I never felt that we were united, my fat and me, until I walked through that Rice House door.

"It's funny because the moment my fat and me became one, I really started to lose weight. I wasn't fighting with anything, I was just on the Rice Diet eating rice and fruit. It was a simple yet profound change. Something just shifted and I knew that I could get to goal weight and my life would never be the same. I accepted all of this like it was laid out in front of me. Lost twenty-five pounds my first month on program.

"I wasn't angry anymore. I wasn't as loud. I was in the process of becoming. I didn't know what I was to ultimately become, but I knew it was better than what I had been.

"My husband and children came to visit me for a weekend after I had been on program for three months. I wouldn't let them come any sooner because I didn't want to break my routine and potentially slow down my weight loss. They were just stunned by the changes. Of course I was much thinner—probably sixty pounds—but I had a different personality too. I think it frightened everybody that I had changed so. Nobody said much that weekend. What could they say? I was cocooning, getting inside myself deeper and deeper. I wasn't transformed yet, but I was on my way. I couldn't explain to my family how I felt. Only another Ricer could understand: your body changes and your heart and mind follow.

"I've always liked the idea that my family can't follow me to the Rice House. Literally speaking, they can, but they can never experience what I do when I am there because they aren't me, they aren't fat, and they aren't Ricers. They could eat the meals that the Rice House offers, but the food would not have the same meaning. To me, everything about the Rice Diet was and is transformative. It is powerful stuff."

After Linda finished talking, I looked up to see the waiter standing patiently by our table. Before I could make a move, Linda handed him her credit card. I thanked her for the interview and the meal, and we walked out to the parking lot together.

Brad Pollock expressed many of the same feelings that Linda had. I interviewed Brad at the Rice House. He was fun to be around and had a gentle humor that he showed off at the dinner table. He teased people, but not in a mean way. Brad was always cordial with everyone. He made sure that each person at the table felt included in the conversation. I liked that about him. He was popular with the Rice House crowd, but didn't isolate himself into a particular group. Even during his interview, he would stop, say hello to people, and acknowledge each person in some way.

After dinner at the Rice House, Brad and I moved to the living room to get away from the noise of the diners. It didn't do any good. Most of the people followed us and sat on the chairs, sofas, and even on the floor to hear Brad's story. His friends were laughing and talking, and Brad motioned for everyone to quiet down. The crowd turned to him expectantly, and he seemed like a preacher as he started to talk. He got up out of his chair and began to pace back and forth. He raised his hands up and out over the crowd and declaimed his story in a booming voice.

Brad Pollock

"I found peace at the Rice House. That was my transforming experience. I started the Diet as one pissed-off fat boy. I was a success by anyone's standards. I had a great and very profitable career, lived in a lovely apartment, took vacations all over the world, and dated models and newscasters. When you have enough money, it doesn't matter how fat you are; at least, that is what I used to believe. Now I know it is not true. Money is just another type of mask, like obesity. They both hide something, and in my case it was my vulnerability. I used money and fat as a defense. I surrounded myself with both of them so I wouldn't have to deal with people on a personal basis. I wheeled and dealed constantly. I thought if I had enough money my obesity would somehow disappear. On the other hand, I ate constantly. If I felt any kind of emotion, either negative or positive, I would eat something.

"I was really a mean, petty, unhappy man. If somebody got in my way at work, I would destroy them. If my girlfriend was unhappy, I would shower her with gifts. If she wanted more, I would dump her and find another one. Even my own mother said I was a mean little bastard!

"At the Rice House, all of that changed. For one thing, I just stopped calling home. Dr. Rosati told me not to phone my mother, my girlfriend, or the office for a month. You got to realize that I was always on the phone. I called the office because I was afraid that I was losing money and somebody was gaining on me, taking over my accounts. I called my mother so I could hear her vent her complaints about what a lousy son I was. Then I would yell at her and hang up. I called my girlfriend for the same reason and to check up on her to make sure she wasn't seeing someone else. I was so jealous. She resented it, but I didn't care.

"Not calling anybody just about killed me, but I did it, and I began to change inside. How I thought about the world changed. The anger just subsided, and the jealousy went away. So what if I lost my job and all of my money? It would be a disaster, but I could survive. So what if my mother died while I was on the Rice Diet? It would be very sad, but life, for me at least, would go on. What if my girlfriend dumped me for my best friend? Again, it would be sad, but not a tragedy. Once you let go of your fears like that, the weight loss just starts to really progress. I learned to let go at the Rice House, and once I did, the weight left too. Of course, I still have to diet constantly, and I exercise daily, but I don't have to carry that extra weight of anger. That's gone."

The Rice House audience was silent. I think many of us were hard pressed to believe that Brad had ever been mean and jealous. After a few moments, people began to get up and move around. Many came over to congratulate Brad and pat him on the shoulder. Brad looked extremely pleased with himself. He got up and walked out of the Rice House with a group of his friends. A few moments later, he came back in and invited me to go with them. I put my things in my car, piled into a minivan with several other Ricers, and went in search of the perfect country-western bar. We found it near Raleigh.

A couple of days after running around with Brad and his friends, I got to know Ellen Mayfield. She was part of Brad's group, although he said he didn't know her well. Ellen described herself as a jealous, vindictive bitch. These were qualities she was very proud of. She never let an insult go unpunished and delighted in the subtle ways she got back at the people she felt had slighted her in some way. Ellen was an attorney from Cincinnati, Ohio, and was single when I interviewed her. I was reluctant to take her interview at first because she had originally thought that my project was a stupid idea. She didn't think the world had any interest in what fat people were all about. After some thought, Ellen changed her mind and decided it was a good idea to talk to me.

We met at the Ninth Street Bakery for coffee. Ellen took the lead in the conversation. I had barely sat down at the table when she began talking. I asked her to hold on a minute and got up to get some coffee. As I was waiting in line for some sugar, Ellen came up and informed me that she had a lot to do and I'd better hurry if I wanted any information from her. Then she stopped abruptly and told me to take my time, that everything was okay. I met her back at the table and drank most of my coffee as Ellen looked around the room and waved to people she knew. When I put down my cup and picked up my notes, Ellen took my free hand and spoke.

Ellen Mayfield

"The Rice House changed me from a mean person to a nice person. You can ask any of my friends; they will all tell you the same thing. I was the meanest, angriest, most aggressive person when I came to Durham. The first couple of months on program nobody would sit next to me because I was so loud and mean. Everything pissed me off: the food was horrible, the participants stupid, and the staff incompetent. The people, I thought, were ignorant. How could so many dumb people be in the world? Also, how could there be so many fat people? I was fat, sure, but I was not *that* fat; at least that is what I told myself. That is really how I felt. I thought everyone was insane. And the doctors! No matter what kind of pain or illness I had, their only response was to tell me to eat rice and fruit. I thought I was going to die on the Rice Diet. Instead, I learned how to live.

"The thing about the Rice Diet is, behavior precedes thought. You change your behavior and the mind follows. Dr. Kempner used to say that, and I thought he was full of shit, but he was right. The other programs probe down to the underlying feelings of why you are fat and try behavior modification. The Rice House doesn't care what you think or how you feel; they just want you to get thin, and fast. I wanted to leave, but a little voice inside me told to stay. The Rice House was my last shot at thinness.

"After a while, the other participants didn't appear as dumb as they had before. The doctors seemed astute, and the food tasted delicious. Of course, when you are starving to death, just about anything tastes good. At first I thought everything around me was changing, but then I realized it was me.

"The thinner I got, the more I changed. It was sort of disorienting at first. I was so used to the old me, the fat me, the angry me. I didn't know how to just be. I learned that at the Rice House. It is okay to just be me."

When she finished, Ellen bought me another cup of coffee, this one to go, and I drove her to her apartment. Two days later, I received a thank-you note in the mail from her. It was the first and only one I got from someone I interviewed.

Kelly Bararrares was a child of the Rice House. At seventeen, she was the youngest person I met on the Rice Diet. I didn't see her much at meals; she had a problem getting to places on time. I didn't see her at weigh-in because she liked to sleep late. She showed up for all the Rice House meetings, looking for something to do that night. There was always a group of Ricers having a party or going to the movies or to some event at Duke. Kelly didn't seem to have a lot of friends. I suppose it was because there wasn't anybody her age around. She did go out with a few of the guys, but didn't seem close to anyone. I met Kelly on the steps of the Rice House for our first informal chat. She wanted to talk to me, but felt she didn't have any insight into diet culture because she was young and not an old-time Ricer. I wanted to talk to Kelly for that very reason—she was younger than most of the people I interviewed, and I thought she would perhaps have a different perspective than the other dieters. She agreed to think about it, but didn't give me a specific time.

One evening in August, a bunch of us decided to go the Starlite drive-in theater on Geer Street. It is the last drive-in in Durham, perhaps the last drive-in on earth, and it is the only one that I have ever been to that is adjacent to a gun shop. You can see a movie and purchase ammo all in one trip. Kelly was part of the group that came along, and she agreed to tell me her story. As we sat in the swings in the kiddie play area in front of the faded screen, gnats and mosquitoes were buzzing all around us, and I could hear crickets and other bugs in the grass. I wondered if my tape recorder and paper could withstand the heat and humidity. I wondered if I could. While the sweat poured off Kelly's face, she swung higher and started talking.

Kelly Bararrares

"I left childhood behind and became an adult at the Rice House, and it is all because of the Rice Diet. I was such a shitty little princess that nobody could stand me. I felt that the entire world owed me a favor, and I thought I should have everything I wanted. My parents did give me everything, but I think they did it because they just wanted me to leave them alone. I was a total brat growing up. I respected nobody and was always getting into other people's stuff and stealing anything I wanted. I got busted when I was twelve years old for stealing a hair clip from Macy's department store. I didn't need it, I just wanted it, and I didn't care if I paid for it or not. I used to steal from my friends and their parents all the time. I used to baby-sit, and I would steal stuff from the houses: necklaces, watches, just stupid stuff like that. I would also go through other people's drawers just to see what they had. I took everything my mom owned. She had nothing to herself. If she bought a tube of lipstick, then I wanted that tube. If she bought perfume, I wanted that perfume too. She would buy two of everything and give me one, but I wanted hers, not mine. I wanted what everyone else had.

"My parents dragged me from one shrink to another. I kept getting kicked out of schools for stealing, or selling drugs, or beating up some kid because he called me fat. I was so mad and jealous all the time. I was mad at the world because it would not cater to me.

I was mad at God and my mother because they made me fat. My mom was always fat, so I blamed her for my weight problems. In fact, I blamed her for everything. My parents had me on all kinds of diet programs. They would even go with me to the meetings and my mom would prepare these low-fat meals. I hated their involvement. I hated that we would all exercise together. I'm sure the neighbors really laughed at seeing all of our fat asses hanging over the bicycle seats as we pedaled around the neighborhood. I just wanted my parents to stay out of my life. I was so embarrassed by them. I didn't want them around at all.

"As a last resort, my grandmother sent me to the Rice House. I weighed almost three hundred pounds at the time, and I was fifteen years old. I hated the Rice House because they didn't give me enough to eat. I tried to explain to the staff that I was not like the other fat people there; I deserved more food. They just ignored me. I lost two hundred pounds in Durham, and it changed my whole outlook. Now I am grateful to God, my parents, and the Rice Diet for making me realize that this is my life and I am totally responsible for everything I do. I shape my own destiny; not God, and not my mom, but me."

I was blown away by Kelly's testimony. It amazed me that this kid had it figured out. I could take lessons from her. I too had felt angry and frustrated for most of my life, and it amazed me that, through weight loss, people could also lose those feelings. Kelly and I stayed outside and tried to watch the movie, but the bugs won, and we went back to the van. We didn't stay to see the end of the movie. It was too hot to keep the windows up and too buggy to put them down.

When we got back to the Rice House, I thanked Kelly for the interview and told her that we would get together again sometime. She smiled and nodded and walked to her car.

Jeff Peacock went from fat to fit on the Rice Diet. Jeff is a thirty-year-old medical student at Duke University originally from Boulder, Colorado. I met Jeff at the track at Duke University. He agreed to talk with me for a few minutes between laps. Jeff ran backward because he believed that it developed his hamstrings. I watched him go round and round the track backward for at least twenty laps. He never turned back once.

Finally, he stopped and I waved to him to come on over. His face was beet red, and he couldn't speak. For a moment, I was afraid that he would drop dead of a heart attack. We walked over to the steps and sat down, and after a few minutes he was able to get his breathing under control. His face returned to its pre-exercise color as he huffed out his words.

Jeff Peacock

"Everything about me changed for the better at the Rice House. I was around 160 pounds overweight and had been so throughout high school and college. I weighed two hundred pounds in sixth grade. As long as I can remember, I was fat. As an obese child, I was the last guy to be picked for any team. Who would want a fat kid to play with them? I was fat, wore glasses, and had asthma. What could be worse? Nobody picked me for anything. I was the quintessential geek. I was good in math and science. Why wouldn't I be? All I did was study because I had no social life. Nobody would go out with me or be my friend.

"When I showed up at the Rice House, I was no longer alone. There were a lot of fat guys just like me, except at the Rice House it was no big deal. I didn't have to suck in my gut all the time and hold my breath like I did at home, because at the Rice House everyone had a big gut. I could finally breathe and relax. I made friends at the Rice House, both male and female. But the thing that truly changed was my attitude about exercise.

"I had always believed that I was exercise impaired. I couldn't run or catch a ball or swing a racket. I could swing a golf club, but I couldn't even walk a nine-hole course. I thought of myself as this huge, lumbering, inept fool. At the Rice House, nobody criticized me for this, and I was picked for teams. I played volleyball, racquetball, tennis, and every other sport you can name. Of course, I wasn't very good at any of them, but it didn't matter. The important thing was that I was moving and playing sports and enjoying every minute of it.

"After I lost about sixty pounds I moved to a motel seven miles from the Rice House. I would walk to the Rice House in the morning, then go to the track at Duke and run around it until I felt like my heart would explode. As I kept losing weight, I started playing more and more sports. I took up every sport imaginable, and I now jog nine miles every day except Sunday. I am studying sports medicine in school and hope to open up my own clinic one day. If it wasn't for the Rice Diet, I wouldn't know how it feels to be fit."

Jeff finished the five minutes he'd promised me and went back to the track. This time he ran with great leaping strides, as though he was cresting imaginary hurdles. I thought about getting on the track with him and running a lap or two just to show him (and myself) that I could do it. I thought better of it and left him alone on the track.

My rites of passage weren't as clear cut as those of my interviewees. My changes were more subtle, but just as powerful. I didn't know how angry I had been or how nervous I'd appeared to others until I went to a doctor's appointment. I had been on the Rice Diet for approximately four months at that point and hadn't seen that doctor since the first day I started the Diet. When I went in for my second appointment, the receptionist told me that she noticed how much weight I'd lost and how I had changed. To her I was no longer the anxious, fidgety, nervous patient of four months ago. Instead, I was calm. Friends also told me that I was not as high-strung as I used to be.

My physical rite of passage came one evening when I took a bubble bath. I was lying in the lavender-scented water when my hand ran over something hard and unfamiliar. The next morning I asked Dr. Newborg to feel the lump in my chest. I knew I had cancer. It was a hard little knot. She assured me that it was not a lump and I didn't have cancer; instead, I had discovered my own sternum. I had never felt it before. After that, I found all kinds of new things: collarbones, hipbones, and even a rib or two. Everything about me was changing.

seven

Durham as Sexual Paradise

When in Durham, united with others like us, we may go through another type of passage—a sexual one. Many of us who come to Durham leave behind significant others. Our intentions are to lose weight and go home to our loved ones as quickly as possible—the same people we always were, but looking and feeling better. We intend to be faithful, but once in Durham, a powerful shift takes place. We meet people who are truly like us. They look like us, act like us, and think like us. We can let our defenses down and become our true selves.

Durham can be a lonely place for dieters. New in town, we do not have the familiar comfort of family and friends. And the biggest comforter of all—food—is banished from our lives. There is no one to turn to except other dieters. Also, rapid weight loss brings in a new element: sexual power. Away from husbands, wives, and the obligations of long-term relationships, Ricers are free to develop their sexual identities, and some even change their sexual preferences.

Ricers see the same people over and over, at least three times a day for meals at the Rice House. Dieters can get very close to each other in a short amount of time. Relationships can flare up and die overnight, or they can take root and last a lifetime.

Sylvia Slossberg believes Durham is the biggest singles bar on earth. I met Sylvia, a seventy-year-old jewelry designer, at a gem show. I was there looking for a replacement piece for a topaz ring. Sylvia was looking for ideas. I approached her and asked her straight out if she was a Ricer. Everything about her shouted Ricer—her clothes, her jewelry, her car, and her accent. She was delighted to give me her life story, and I was thrilled to interview her. Sylvia was fun. She took me to a private club somewhere near Cary, where we had an elegant dinner of Norwegian salmon and pasta with cream sauce. Sylvia requested everything on the side—her salad dressing, the cream for the pasta. Even the capers that accompanied the salmon were in their own separate bowl. She didn't eat any of the dressing or capers. For dessert we had berries with clotted cream. Sylvia ate a berry or two, then put the bowl aside.

I had never seen a more beautiful woman than Sylvia Slossberg. She was as old as my mother, but she could have passed for my sister. There wasn't a hard line about her, not in her face or body. Everything—hair, eyes, and body—was soft and round. She was not fat, not to me, but she was cushy and had a lushness about her. She was very happy, and her personality filled the room.

People at other tables turned to glance at us. They probably thought that Sylvia was a retired movie star. She would nod her head slightly toward each admirer, and they would turn away, pleased and embarrassed. I watched her lovely hands smooth away the imaginary wrinkles in the pristine tablecloth. Without looking up at me, Sylvia began talking.

Sylvia Slossberg

"Durham is the most fantastic place I have ever seen. The whole town is one huge singles bar. Where else could a woman my age find so many lovers—young ones, at that. I tell all of my friends and their daughters and granddaughters that if they want to get married, they should come to Durham and go on a diet program. I have been coming to Durham since the 1960s, and it's still as exciting as it was back then. People will try to tell you different, but Durham has a lot going on. People always look back in longing at the past, but Durham is still the place of action to me. I met all of my husbands at the Rice House. Dr. Kempner used to refer to me as the lady with the wash-and-wear wedding dress! And it was true. I love Ricers. They are the best husbands in the world for around six months or so. Unfortunately, they are a transient bunch and not much for long-term commitment, but they are so much fun in the beginning.

"When I first went on the Rice Diet I wasn't even that fat—maybe twenty pounds over my ideal weight—but I thought of myself as extremely obese. This was the 1960s, and everybody was thin. Clothes were short and tight, and I wanted to look good. The Rice House was the place to be. The air was just filled with excitement and sexual desire. You could smell it.

"You can't control all your appetites at the same time. It's impossible. You can control food or sex, but not both. I had all those horny men at the Rice House, and all these young studs from Duke who wanted to know if the Rice Diet was some kind of aphrodisiac, which, of course, it is. God, I love Durham.

"I met my first husband the first day on program. He was this big ol' Texan with a huge gut on him. Initially, I was turned off by him because he was as wide as he was tall, and so full of bullshit. He would tease me all the time about politics. I am a Democrat, and he was a Republican, and he would rib me about that. Then one night he just put the moves on me, made a play for me, but I recoiled. I didn't tell him that his weight scared me off, but he knew. He wasn't offended at all. He just said, 'Honey, you can count to ten and stand anything, can't you?' And I could, and I did. I grew very fond of him and we were married six months after we met. He was a very rich man. He died two years into the marriage, but he left me a lot of money. As he told me once, it is better to be rich 'because there is nothing like farting through silk.' He was right.

"My other husbands were pretty much cut from the same cloth. All of them were obese, ill, rich, and lonely. Some of them were married when I met them, but that didn't stop them or me. Durham is different. The rules that apply at home don't apply there. Also, when people lose weight and get healthy and feel better about themselves, they just go on the prowl. The other women at the Rice House used to call me the Barracuda. They thought I was only there to take away their supply of boyfriends. You see, I *wasn't* as fat as the other women, and I was more fun."

Sylvia finished talking and told me it was time to go, that she had another appointment. I imagined that it was with a lover she had tucked away somewhere. We walked to our cars, and she pulled a pale silk scarf out of her bag and wrapped it around her head so that the ends of it trailed across her throat and down her back. It made me think of something Audrey Hepburn would have done in a movie with Cary Grant. I waited until her car was out of the parking lot, then got in my car and drove back to Durham.

Abby Felcher also found Durham a sexual playground and as exciting a dating scene for older women as Sylvia did. We met at my house to chat, and Abby regaled me with juicy tidbits about fellow Ricers and their sexual escapades. After a while, I got out my notes and tape recorder, and Abby fiddled with her artificial nails as she started talking.

Abby Felcher

"Durham is incredible for me. Sex is abundant and without any long-term complications. Relationships are just the way I like them, brief and to the point. I knew what Durham was like before I ever got here. I had heard the stories about wild parties where people went naked. I knew they had to be true, because what else are you going to do in Durham on a diet? You can't eat, so you might as well screw. I asked the old man [Dr. Kempner] once, how many calories did I burn up during sexual intercourse? He told me that the average person uses approximately one hundred and fifty calories during sex. Kempner didn't bat an eye when he told me. I am sure hundreds of Ricers have asked him that question. I was disappointed that I only burned that small amount of calories. Still, it was better than nothing.

"Immediately after starting the program, I met this gentleman who had been on the Diet for a couple of weeks. He was a few years younger than I, but that didn't seem to matter. We hit it off right away, and we started going out for coffee after dinner. It was no big thing, and we went with a group of other Ricers, but it was clear to everyone that I liked him and he liked me. Soon, we were going off on our own. A couple of times we skipped dinner and even the morning weigh-in. Soon we were being talked about at the Rice House. I supposed I should have been embarrassed because I am of a certain age and I was behaving foolishly—and he was married. But I didn't feel one single moment of embarrassment or regret. I didn't care what anyone thought of me. I felt happy! I felt really happy and alive. It struck me when I was with him, how lonely and bored and on autopilot I had been in my marriage. Nothing thrilled me, nothing turned me on. I just went through the motions of being involved in my own life.

"All that time I thought it was me. I didn't think of myself as a sexual being because I was old and fat, and to the world, I was nothing at all. My husband didn't care for me sexually. When we were together he told me that he was attracted to me, but not as attracted as he would be to someone thinner than I. That did it for me. I never looked at him the same way, and when he initiated sex, I froze. I used to blame myself because I was the one who was fat. Perhaps on a subconscious level I was remaining fat because I didn't want to be with my husband. Frankly, I didn't like him. I resented him because he had this conditional love for me. He only liked me thin. If I was thin enough, he would provide me with sex. If I was too fat for him, he would punish me by withholding sex. I got to the point where I didn't care one way or another.

"When I met my lover at the Rice House, something that had been frozen inside of me for many, many years thawed. I became a sexual being again. I was like a teenager. I could hardly wait to get him alone. We were holding hands and kissing in the parking lot for God's sake. It was an amazing time. It wasn't love at all, it was sex and freedom and just plain joy of being alive. I used to walk around his apartment naked—not a thing on—and I felt so beautiful. Hey, I was old and fat, but to him I was fantastic, and he made me feel that way.

"It didn't last long. Soon he had to go home to his wife and family, and I understood it. 'No regrets' was our motto. You learn that real quick at the Rice House. Nothing lasts. It didn't take me long to find someone else in Durham, and it was just as great as the first time. I love Durham. It is where I was awakened sexually. I woke up, and I stayed awake."

I knew what she meant. I too woke up in Durham. I had always considered myself a sexually liberated and fulfilled woman, but it wasn't until I met someone at the Rice House that I felt beautiful, powerful, and free. I smiled to myself and Abby nodded. She knew what I was thinking. We talked on into the night, and somewhere in the middle of it, we raised our glasses to lovers past, present, and future.

Cindy Sitco found sexual freedom also. Cindy and I went to the movies one night out of sheer boredom. The movie was boring too, so we walked across the parking lot to a Dairy Queen. It's interesting how everywhere in the diet capital of the world you are within walking distance of some forbidden place. We split a small cup of nonfat vanilla yogurt. Cindy took tiny bites and savored every one of them. After we were finished, she looked around to make sure no one was close enough to hear her remarks. She kicked me playfully under the table and, in a quiet voice, started talking.

Cindy Sitco

"I had been at the Rice House for a while and had lost a significant amount of weight, maybe seventy pounds. I had made a lot of friends in Durham and had established a life. I ate all my meals at the Rice House, walked every morning in Duke Forest with a bunch of Ricers, worked three afternoons a week for an accounting firm in Durham on a contracted basis, and went to Duke Chapel church services on Sunday mornings. I had a life like the one I left in Kansas City, but I was thinner and alone in Durham. I left my boyfriend back home. He did come to visit once, but it was uncomfortable having him around me at the Rice House. It was jarring. He didn't belong there.

"I had just weighed in and gotten off the scales when this incredibly handsome man walked in. I looked up and caught his eye, and something was exchanged between us. From that moment on, we were inseparable. It was his first day on program, and when he sat down at the table all of these women were preening and fluttering all around him, but all he saw was me. I was so flattered and a bit overwhelmed and off-kilter. I was the one who usually initiated a relationship. Now the tables were turned. He courted me. He really did court me in the old-fashioned sense of the word. He sent me flowers and notes and left little gifts on my doorstep. He left long messages on my answering machine. He had this lovely baritone voice and would sing messages on my machine from Broadway musicals. I love musicals; he knew that, and he had all these playbills from the great ones. I still have a couple in my box of Ricer mementos. He even wrote me a poem. God, it sounds foolish now, but it was so much fun, and I had such a crush. At my age, I was having a crush on somebody. It was thrilling.

"Within a week we were lovers. He knocked on my door after dinner one evening, and I opened it and we just embraced and went down to the floor and just stayed there for a couple of hours. It was unbelievable the passion we felt for each other. Later on, we made it to my bedroom and continued our lovemaking.

"This went on for a couple of months. I didn't think once about food or eating or even about losing weight. I didn't think anything about my boyfriend back home. I didn't answer his phone calls or anything. That part of my life was over as far as I was concerned. All I thought about was my new lover. Then one night we were supposed to go out somewhere, to a movie I think, and he just didn't show up. I called his apartment and the phone rang and rang. The answering machine didn't pick up. I drove to his place and saw his car. I went to the door, but nobody answered. I left a note on his car asking him to call me the moment he got in. I was too restless to go home, so I went to the bar at the Sheraton. I never went there before. Why should I? I wasn't looking to pick up anybody because I was already in love. He was there with another woman. Actually, he was with three other women, and they were all laughing and talking. When he looked up and saw me, all the color drained out of his face. He looked deflated. Even his body sagged. I just turned to him and raised up my glass in a cheers salute and nodded my head. I forced myself to stay a few minutes. I even chatted with the bartender and pretended I was happy. And then the weirdest thing happened. I realized I *was* happy. I was angry, hurt, and extremely jealous at first, but all those emotions passed quickly, and I turned around and genuinely smiled at him. He smiled and shrugged his magnificent shoulders. We did have great sex, and I guess the effects of it lasted a long time. Never underestimate the power of a great lay. I felt good, free, and strong. Besides, this is Durham. Relationships fade quickly and nothing lasts, and sometimes that's a good thing."

Cindy stopped and got up for another cup of yogurt. This time she got vanilla and chocolate swirl. I doubted that it was the non-fat variety. All of the sex talk must have perked up her appetite. It certainly did mine. I got up and bought myself a chocolate and vanilla swirl topped with M&Ms. I would regret this indulgence later, but it felt so good and wicked at the time. It was hard to believe that Cindy could be passionate about anything. I always thought her contained and depressed. At some point in her life, she had been happy. As I watched her drive away, I wished her happiness in the future and a lot more fun.

Reva Collins found true love at the Rice House. I met Reva, a forty-four-year-old acquisitions editor for a major press, at breakfast at the Rice House. I told her about my project, and she agreed to meet later in the day at my house. Over rice crackers and Red Zinger tea, she told me about love at the Rice House. I liked Reva a lot. She was one of those big, beautiful women, with an abundant spirit and a great soul. She seemed perfectly content and at peace with herself and the world around her. I envied her beauty and her poise. She swore a lot, but it sounded elegant when she did it.

Reva Collins

"My initiation into the Rice Diet was a sexual one. Durham is a fat girl's paradise, and the Rice House is the biggest singles bar in the world. Blue Chips, Crisco Disco, and all the other clubs that have Fat Night were a dream come true for me. I never wanted to leave.

"I knew what this town was all about the first time I got here. I was fat as a hog, and all kinds of men were hitting on me, asking me out, slipping me notes—and this was before I even got to the Rice House. I was in line at a Chinese carry-out getting my Last Supper right before I started the Diet, and some stranger came up and gave me his business card and asked me out that very evening. They like fat girls in Durham. I stayed at the Sheraton, and it was full of men on the make. There were chubby chasers galore around the bar just waiting for someone like me to show up. And I knew when I walked into the Sheraton that it was my lucky day. I knew Durham was going to be fun.

"I had had relationships before with several people—both male and female. When you are a certain size it is just accepted by the general population that you are either a dyke or a slut, maybe both. Being fat, I settled for less in relationships. I knew I was settling for less, and it pissed me off, but I settled anyway. Everybody wanted to fuck me, but they wanted to do it after they dropped their girlfriends off. I did it too. What did I care? Most of my serious relationships were with married men—married men who were married to thin women. That is the way it goes. A man once told me this—it's like eating chicken all the time; you start craving steak. I guess I was the red meat that married men craved.

"I started the Rice Diet with a chip on my shoulder and with the attitude that I didn't give a shit about anybody, especially some guy. I rejected people before they could reject me. I know shrinks would say that I was masking some deeper insecurity, but that wasn't it at all. Deep down, I really didn't care. I was living the existential life. I was passionless and pain-free.

"Quietly, almost without my knowledge, I began to change. I woke up feeling expectant. I would go to the Rice House and sit at a table and this buoyancy would come over me. I would feel like I was going to float right out of the room. As my body decreased, my heart increased. I started to feel everything—happiness, joy, and tremendous sorrow. I cried for a month when I first started the Rice Diet. It was a horrible deep aching sorrow that surfaced. The more weight I lost, the more feelings I got. I just cried and cried. I cried in exhilaration that I was getting thin, and I cried for my old lost self.

"I found love at the Rice House. I found the kind of love that I thought only happened in books. I was sitting at the farthest table from the door on a Sunday morning, and this man walked in and sat right across from me and asked, 'What's your story?' If it had been anyplace but the Rice House, I would have told him to fuck off, but instead, I told him my life story. And he told me his. His was so similar to mine it was scary. He had a history of relationships with older married women, and I had a history of being with older married men. We started being together as often as possible, and as soon as we could we rented an apartment a mile from the Rice House. We made love every moment we could, and it was the most blissful kind of lovemaking because we were so connected. We were both fat and used to hiding the obvious, but together we could be ourselves and enjoy our bodies. He didn't have to worry about sucking in his gut all the time, and I didn't have to worry about the placement of my body. Really, when you are fat you worry about how you drape—is there a fold here, is a part flopping over there, is the cellulite compressed and looking even worse than usual? There was none of that. We were just two people—two normal people deeply in love."

Reva looked wistful and turned away for a moment. I wondered if she ever saw him, her great love, or had he just drifted away like most Ricers? She turned back and was her usual composed self. We left the Rice House together and drove to Duke Forest for a morning hike. Reva didn't say much and neither did I. We just enjoyed our walk in the woods.

Men, even more than women, can find Durham a sexual paradise. Women on diet programs outnumber men four to one. A single, reasonably healthy man is the center of attention at the Rice House. The man who commanded the most attention at the Rice House was Stephen Conners. He was the darling of all the women at the Rice House. I thought he, more than any other male Ricer, would know if Durham was a sexual paradise.

When I approached him for an interview, I was prepared to tape him right then and there. Instead, he suggested we meet for dinner at the Magnolia Grill in Durham. The Grill was his favorite restaurant in the area, and he felt that I too should experience its pleasures. I was intimidated by Stephen because he was very powerful, rich, handsome, and self-possessed. Unlike other men I have interviewed, he didn't demand certain limitations on the conversation or set up any kind of parameters for the interview. He let things happen. He was not anxious or demanding or even particularly charming. He was just self-confident. It was disarming.

I was on time for my dinner with Stephen. It didn't take me much time to get ready because I had only one outfit that was appropriate for the Magnolia Grill. It was a loaner black dress from a fellow Ricer with a pair of stiletto pumps she'd urged me to wear. Unfortunately, I had to park some distance from the restaurant. I hobbled up to the entrance in my borrowed shoes, hoping no one had seen me. Stephen was already at a table, and the waiter led the way. I sat down, and Stephen poured me a glass of wine. For dinner he ordered several appetizers, and I sampled all of them. It was a good meal. As the waiter cleared away our plates, Stephen motioned for two coffees, turned to me and began.

Stephen Conners

"I love Durham for so many reasons and one is the availability of pretty young girls who want to sleep with an old man like me. Durham is a sexual paradise, especially for men. There are many more women than men in Durham, and they are all lonely and away from home. Some of them are on their own for the first time in their lives. Not all of them are really fat either. They wouldn't be considered fat in another era, but now I guess the style is to be skinny. To me, they all look good. They are very much aware of their appearance. After all, they are here to lose weight, so they are conscious of how they look. They make an effort to wear stylish clothes, get their hair and nails done, have their makeup perfect. Most of the girls here are smart, educated, and successful, but when it comes to men, they don't know much. Many of them have never had decent relationships with any man in their lives, not even their fathers. Some of them, I guess, are looking for father figures. I fit the bill. I've dated many a young girl at the Rice

House, and nobody thought it was a big deal. In any town other than Durham, I would have probably been arrested, but in Durham it's okay. I used to go out with a whole gaggle of young girls to bars, restaurants, the movies, clubs, and such. I would feel so good walking into a place with these young girls hanging all over me. It was quite flattering. I had sex all the time, and more often than not I had sex with two or three of them at once.

"It wasn't always that way. Before the Rice Diet, before I lost weight and got my health back, I couldn't have sex, didn't have sex for years. You know, I figured, what the hell, I'm old and who would want to have sex with me anyhow? Not my wife, that's for sure. Not any women I knew. No, they just saw me as a sick old man. I *was* sick too, with diabetes, heart problems, and just plain old age. At the Rice House, it all changed. I went off my medications, quit smoking, lost weight, started exercising regularly, all the things they told me to do for years but I never did. At the Rice House, I just started doing them, and I got to feel better, and women were beginning to find me attractive and look upon me as a sexual partner. What an ego boost! Back home everyone treated me like I was already dead, and in Durham I had young girls grabbing my hand under the table at dinner. Amazing.

"I fell in love with one of them. I was at least thirty years her senior, but she didn't seem to mind. She was so determined that we would be lovers. She followed me everywhere, even asked to go on errands with me. She wrote me poems. She was a sweet girl and very lonely. Her body was soft and round and so young. She hung on my every word. She worshipped me. It was all so flattering, but I tried not to take it to heart. Still, her wide-open desire was such a turn-on to me that I finally gave in. She literally took me in the dressing room of a department store at Northgate Mall. Jesus, it was wonderful. I wasn't even sure I could manage to perform, but I did. She fell asleep in my car on the way home. I must have looked upon her sleeping face for twenty minutes before I woke her. I just drove around. Drove all the way to Chapel Hill and back. I didn't want to disturb her. We were lovers for a whole summer, until she met some young tennis player and took up with him. She once asked me if there was ever a time when a person got past the need for sexual desire. I told her yes, you reach a point when all passion is spent. It is not true. You are passionate until the day you die—ask any man at the Rice House."

Stephen finished his story, took a sip of his coffee, and looked at me over his cup. I looked back at him and felt my face getting red. I could see how someone could fall for him. Maybe I was falling myself. The delicious food, the wine, the coffee, and his story all seemed to enhance the atmosphere. He paid the bill when it came, but didn't get up. I stayed in my seat for a while wondering what it would be like to be with him. After a while, I stood up and so did he. We walked arm in arm to my car on the premise that I might fall off my high heels or that the wine had gone to my head. Actually, I just wanted to touch his arm and feel his presence. He kissed me on my forehead and said goodnight. As I pulled away and began to drive down the street, I turned my head to see if he was still watching. Stephen waved to me and smiled.

David Ramsey found heartbreak in Durham. I met David at the Rice House for the interview and found out that I had known him when I lived in Virginia. David was from the same town. We had lived on the same block and nodded to each other on the way to the subway each morning.

It seemed funny that I would meet my former neighbor at the Rice House. David and I had coffee at Elmo's Diner, but first he made me walk to Duke Chapel and back with him. I suppose he was testing to see if I was really a Ricer and could keep up with him. I barely made it.

David got to Elmo's first. I was a good two blocks behind him. When I finally made it to the parking lot, he was waiting for me on the steps. We got a table and ordered glasses of iced tea. It was too noisy in the diner to hear each other talk, so we drained our tea and walked to Duke's east campus. We sat on the grass. All around us students were reading, sleeping, and sunning themselves. David leaned back on his elbows and looked up to the sky as he spoke.

David Ramsey

"Durham is where I left my heart. My heart was healed in Durham, and my heart was broken there too. I have heart disease and have had bypass surgery as well as several other procedures. I have been on a variety of medications that produced more complications than cures. The Rice Diet eliminated the progression of my disease. I can breathe without feeling that somebody is standing on my chest, I am off most of my medication, and I have lived longer than my cardiologist said I would. So you see, Durham and the Rice Diet healed my damaged heart. Physically, my heart is better; emotionally, it still hurts.

"I fell in love at the Rice House for the first time in my life. I know that sounds trite for a man my age, but it is true. I fell in love with this beautiful girl who shall remain nameless. She looked like some kind of goddess out of an old painting. She was statuesque and gorgeous. She wasn't thin by a long shot, but she was beautiful. She had this long bundle of hair that was the color of wheat, and the whitest skin I had ever seen. She was also a lot younger than I. She sat down in the chair next to me in the dining room, and that was it. I was speechless. As long as I live I will never forget the moment I saw her.

"One thing led to another, and soon we were living together. For a couple of months everything was perfect. We had a little apartment, ate all our meals at the Rice House, and walked all over Durham. We were both losing weight like mad. Her parents heard about what was going on and flew to Durham to put a stop to it. Here was this older, married man shacking up with their daughter, who was in Durham to diet, not to fall in love. Once they met me and saw us together, they sort of relented and just let things be. They went back home, and we continued on together.

"One day, out of the blue, my wife came to visit. Things were a little tense. Here I was sitting at the table in the Rice House with my wife on one side and my girlfriend on the other. Everyone knew what was going on, but nobody said anything. The Rice House is that kind of place. Whatever goes on at the Rice House stays at the Rice House. It is an unwritten law.

"I eventually told my wife about my girlfriend. I asked for a divorce. There was no point in prolonging a marriage that was empty. My wife said we should give it some time and see how things went. I agreed. I gave it some time. I went home and my girlfriend went back to her family. We were supposed to meet back in Durham in three months. I stayed in Durham four months waiting for her to appear, but she never did. I've sent registered letters which have all been returned. I even flew out to visit her parents, who said that she didn't want to see me.

"I go back to the Rice House from time to time to keep my heart disease at bay and to see if anyone has heard from her. Now and then, someone will say that they saw her somewhere, but nobody is very specific about it. I have given up trying to find her. I just hope that someday she returns to the Rice House."

David finished his story, laid back, and covered his eyes with his arm. I didn't know want to say. I wanted to comfort him somehow, but couldn't think of anything appropriate. I thanked him for sharing his experiences with me and told him I hoped that she really would come back one day. I left him lying on the ground and walked back to the Rice House.

Many of the people I talked to had found romance in Durham. Sometimes it was merely sexual and brief, and sometimes it was sexual and brief but extremely powerful and transforming. A few found true love at the Rice House, and some found rejection and disappointment. All of them found a sense of acceptance and passion that they hadn't discovered anywhere else. I knew what they were talking about. I've felt what they've felt. I knew what it was like to settle for less all of your life and then wind up in Durham surprised to be in love, and I knew where love could and couldn't take you.

I was single when I was at the Rice House. I had a long-term relationship, but my boyfriend was back home, and I was lonely in Durham: lonely, bored, and extremely restless. I was looking for something—or someone—to occupy my time, to entertain me, to distract me from those troubling thoughts of forbidden food. I was looking for a good time.

I dated furiously at the Rice House. Dated everyone I met. I went everywhere with everyone and enjoyed every minute of it. It was fun dating Ricers because they were just as bored and restless as I was and wanted to go places and do things. Money was no object, and neither was time, because all there is in Durham is excess time. You can't eat, so you have to fill up your days and nights with other pursuits.

Ricers are the perfect dates. They are perfect in a 1950s sort of way: very charming, gallant, and reserved. They pick you up in their shiny clean cars, their skin smelling of soap, and they bring gifts and flowers, and sometimes plane tickets. They remember every occasion and even send notes to your mother. Then they go home, and the fairytale ends until another Prince Charming arrives at the Rice House—a large one, yes, but still a prince.

I fell in love three times at the Rice House. Once with an old man, once with a boy, and once with a fellow who, in retrospect, seemed straight out of a romance novel. I loved the excitement, the crushes, the anticipation, the yearning of falling in love. I loved the desire, the way my heart pounded when he walked into the room—all that stuff I should have felt in high school, but didn't. At the Rice House, I felt like a prom queen. Every Ricer that I dated made me feel beautiful and desirable and even adorable just the way I was. And I never felt fat. Of course, I was fat and still am, but I never felt fat with a Ricer. I felt free in every sense of the word. I felt liberated. I had lots of attention, lots of fun, and a little bit of heartache. I have often surmised that it was the lack of food—perhaps low blood sugar—that made my senses so enhanced. I remember every look, every touch, every kiss, and each goodbye.

Sex and love are easy to find in Durham. All of us find them. We are uprooted from our daily lives, and restraints like marriages or relationships seem far away. Weight, health, age, and attractiveness don't seem to be barriers in Durham. Seeing the same people three times a day, seven days a week, all going through the same program, experiencing the same feelings, and having the same needs leads to the development of intense emotions. Deep attachments develop quickly. This emotionality can appear reckless to some, especially those at home who just don't understand what is happening to their loved ones in Durham. But to us, it is liberating. We are free to experience everything, and to find out what we are made of, to find out who we are. During this heady period, we believe that nothing can touch us and we will reach goal weight, be cured of our lifelong obesity, and start a new life. We are so in love and so happy about our weight loss that we don't even get hungry. It is at this exhilarating point in our dieting journey that many of us start experiencing a pang or two of hunger or regret. This is when we begin to be less conscious of the Diet's requirements, and we start to slip and slide back into disorderly eating patterns. Our old habits try to reassert themselves.

eight

Backsliding

Backsliding is the experience of eating off the program or outside the Rice House. Worshippers of the Diet call it sin; others call it picking up salt. The Rice Diet is very low in salt, so any cheating on the Diet is uncovered through the presence of higher sodium levels. Backsliding occurs when we are at low points. We have been on the Diet for several weeks or months, the monotony of eating every meal at the Rice House gets to be too much, and the call of our old love, food, gets stronger and more persistent. Backsliding often occurs when out-of-town guests visit. The temptation to go back to our old ways is overwhelming, and we give in to social pressure and appetite.

When we eat outside the Rice House, it shows up in weight gain and high sodium levels. When I was there, the whole Rice House knew immediately who backslid because the staff publicly displayed sodium count results. The Rice House staff reprimands a backslider, but does not criticize, accepting the sinner but not the sin. Backsliding shows us to be human, and we acknowledge our sin humbly. The Rice House community, in turn, embraces us for our weakness in eating off the program and our strength in showing our humility. Backsliding is part of Ricer initiation.

Sin City, also known as Destruction Alley or Murderer's Row, is a half mile from the Rice House and features fast-food restaurants.

From the sides of the road, Kentucky Fried Chicken, Dunkin' Donuts, Taco Bell, and Golden Corral beckon. Sin City is off-limits, but all of us believe that the businesses here are intended to tempt dieters. Proprietors know we are in town to lose weight, but they also know we are dying to eat something forbidden. The anonymity of the drive-through window appeals to our need for seclusion. It enhances the cheating experience. When we are at our nadir, tired of the strain and commitment of dieting, Sin City beckons.

Men and women backslide differently. When men backslide, they proceed in a grand style and then brag about how much they ate or drank. Male backsliders are angry, yet proud, when they cheat. They are often mad at themselves because they have spent so much time and money to get to Durham and waste it by backsliding, but proud that the Rice House staff cannot dominate them. Men display what they believe to be a healthy defiance by cheating on the Diet from time to time. Through backsliding, they assert their wills against the official will of the Rice House. They defy the authority of the Diet.

Women take a less allegorical and more personal path. We cheat a little bit here and there while on the Diet, a slip rather than an all-out assault. Women tend to accept free samples at the upscale gourmet grocery and specialty stores that surround Durham and Chapel Hill. We feel disobedient and disloyal when we cheat. We explain our backsliding as something beyond our control, something that just comes upon us, rather than as a conscious act. We don't feel proud about backsliding, just foolish and ashamed.

The Rice House staff is well aware of the temptations of food, dieters' weak wills, and their emotional needs. Often a staff member can be found wandering in and out of the popular Ricer hangouts, looking for cheaters. Rumor has it that in the old days, Kempner would prowl Ricer haunts for delinquent dieters, haul them back to the Rice House, and sometimes kick them off the program. Now dieters are admonished for their behavior and encouraged to return to the program immediately.

When we begin the Rice Diet, we tell ourselves and others that we will never cheat. After all, the Rice Diet is the final one for us, and it seems absurd that we would cheat on it. Old-timers nod sagely and chuckle at our fresh enthusiasm. They know better. They have been Ricers for a long time.

Old-timers like to scare and entertain newcomers with popular backsliding stories. These stories function as warnings of the consequences of consuming taboo foods after weeks of existing on pure Rice House food. These stories help keep us on track. They acknowledge the tension between our passion for forbidden food and the consequences of letting our appetite get out of control. Yet going off the Diet is an unavoidable and necessary step. We must learn to accept with grace the human failure of backsliding.

Many backsliding events recounted by the Rice House staff are horror stories of Ricers who backslide so far that they die, or even worse, regain their weight! The Rice House doctors are very aware of the pull of family and job obligations on their patients and present appropriate parables to address these tensions. In his weekly talks, Dr. Rosati, the medical director of the Rice House, often tells the story of a Ricer who almost reached her goal weight, but had to go home due to a family emergency. She told the Rice House staff that she would return to Durham in a couple of weeks, but did not show up. Months later, a fellow Ricer accidentally bumped into her on the street. The Ricer didn't recognize her once thin and happy fellow dieter. The friend, now grossly overweight, looked terrible. The Ricer was shocked, the ex-Ricer was ashamed and slunk away. This is a woman's story, and in it the woman puts her family before herself.

The male horror story ends in death. Dr. Rosati tells this one to warn men to resist the persistent call of business, just as women should resist the pull of family. In this story, a man nearly reached his goal weight, but had to rush home to attend a business crisis. The Rice House doctors pleaded with the man not to leave, because he was not yet cured of his heart disease, but the man returned to the pressures of his job. One night he was very tired and backslid into his old habit of eating food that was bad for his health. Before he was even aware of it, he was eating a lamb chop instead of rice and fruit. He ate and died. That one lamb chop killed him. According to this parable, leaving the Rice House before a permanent change in eating behavior has taken root is deadly, and even one slip off the Diet can kill.

When we fall off of the program and go on a binge, many of us do it in Sin City, whose purpose is to lure weak-willed dieters into the abyss. After one is on a diet program for weeks or months, the call of Sin City gets stronger and stronger.

Bob Hobgood, a retired attorney from Little Rock, Arkansas, had been known to make late-night visits to Sin City. I interviewed him at the Rice House after dinner, and enjoyed talking to him because he gave me his version of the classic Ricer tale of food and sex, the Arnie and Veronica story, a folktale of Ricer culture that I heard from several Dieters.[21] He was fun to be with and relished telling me his own backsliding escapade. I knew Bob cheated because sometimes he didn't show up at the Rice House for weeks, and when he did, he always appeared a little puffier.

On the day of our meeting, Bob was thinner than usual and very proud of it. He informed me that he had lost six pounds in one day and that if he kept up that pace he would reach goal in no time. I nodded and laughed with him. We all promise ourselves that we will lose quickly and at the same rate every day. That never happens. I ate my meal with Bob. We both had the same thing: a bowl of rice with a side of tomato sauce, a banana, and a small bowl of canned peaches. Some Ricers got up and left as I got out my recorder, but others gathered around to hear Bob. His reputation as a storyteller was well known in the community. He pushed his chair back, folded his delicate hands over his big belly and began.

Bob Hobgood

"I have been around the Rice House for many years, and I have heard all of the great old stories about wild Ricers who run amok in Durham. They are standards now and part of diet culture, but who knows if they are really true? I guess it doesn't matter because they sound like something Ricers would do. You know, stories about Ricers who go into a Chinese restaurant and order everything on the right-hand side of the menu, Ricers who go to every restaurant in town and drop a grand at dinner, Ricers who have to be forcibly removed from all-you-can-eat restaurants like Shoney's and Golden Corral. Ricers love to eat more than anything. That's why Durham has so many good restaurants. A Ricer can tell you every meal he ever had or where to get the best pizza, cheesecake, or egg roll. We associate everything with food.

"One famous tale is the Arnie and Veronica story. It still dominates as part of our folklore, and I even read about it in *Esquire* magazine. If you are a Ricer, you probably know this story. When Ricers sit around the front porch after dinner and talk, this is one of the first stories that comes up.

"Arnie was a Ricer and so huge that he had a problem getting women to sleep with him, so he hired a prostitute named Veronica. She came breezing into his room one night with a pink chiffon scarf about her neck. Veronica was just what Arnie ordered. She was sweet, young, professional, and compliant. If he had the money, she would spend the night with him, and Arnie, being a rich Ricer, had the money. Arnie and Veronica made a night of it. He ordered six complete dinners of ribs, cole slaw, tiny taters, pecan pie, and three six-packs of beer from a take-out rib joint. Eating is the foreplay of all fat people. Sex begins with an appetizer. It is a prerequisite for a night of pleasure.

"After dinner they smoked some pot and drank even more beer. Arnie ate in bed (he was too fat to walk) with Veronica, and he was sucking pig fat off his greasy fingers and splattering barbecue sauce all over the place during his feeding frenzy. Veronica didn't seem to mind; in fact, she enjoyed all of his appetites. In the morning, a hung-over Arnie found himself in a blood-soaked (actually barbecue-sauced) bed surrounded by rib bones and one tattered pink scarf. Arnie believed that he had eaten Veronica!

"Now, you can take this story two ways: one, that he actually consumed her, or two, that he had oral sex with her. Being a Ricer, he probably did both. Ricers have strong appetites in every area. This is a great story and depends a lot on the skill of the teller. I heard this story the first day I was on the Diet, and I often tell it to the new people. I like to see the fear and disgust in their eyes. But really, you get so hungry on this diet you could actually commit cannibalism.

"The first time I cheated was at a Taco Bell. Mexican food is the worst possible choice for a cheat because it is loaded with salt. I decided to have just one bean burrito—not a grande, but a regular-sized one. How bad could that be? I was willing to gain a few pounds for the pleasure of tasting that burrito. I had been on the Diet for seventy days. I went to the drive-through window and glanced up at the menu. The next thing I knew I was ordering three burrito supremes, nachos, refried beans, a king-size Pepsi, and everything else on the menu. I actually ordered three from each category. The girl at the window couldn't believe it. I told her I was having a party. What else could I say? Cost me over three hundred dollars. I pulled into the parking lot and spent forty-five minutes just gorging on food. Food was flying all over the car. Thank God I was alone. It felt so good to just fill up like the old days.

"Actually, I never had consumed that much food in one sitting before, but that night I just couldn't stop myself. It was the saltiness that turned on my appetite. After that first bite, I just wanted more and more food. There was food all over me and all over the inside of my car. Even the windows were spattered with food. There was taco sauce, hamburger, and dripping cheese everywhere. I looked like I had been in a bad car wreck. I must have looked like Arnie on the morning after. I went back to my hotel room and became deathly ill. I was sick all night. I didn't show up for weigh-in at the Rice House the next day, or the next three days. Finally, somebody called to see if I was still alive, and I decided to go back in. Nobody was at all surprised that I had backslid. The doctors shook their heads, but didn't say much. Norma, the nurse at the Rice House, told me that it cost me around a grand to backslide when you consider the charges of the medical fees, the Rice House meal fees, rent, and transportation. That amount doesn't even take into consideration the time off work I wasted in Durham not dieting. Cheating is a foolish thing, but it sure feels good.

"Now when I cheat I go to good restaurants. I don't take any of the novice Ricers with me, because I don't want to influence them. I take a bunch of old buddies and we go out and have a dining experience. Sure, I pick up some salt, and it takes me a couple of days to dump the gained weight, but it is worth it. I am human, you know, and man cannot live on rice alone."

After our interview, Bob gave me a ride home. His car smelled of stale sausage biscuits—greasy and yeasty. I didn't say anything about it because I assumed that the cheats were his way of coping. Who was I to judge, anyway: food has always been my way of dealing with things too. Bob knew I noticed the smell, but said nothing. I waved him goodbye and wondered if he was going to stop by McDonald's on his way home.

John Fredrick found temporary comfort in his first cheat in Sin City, just as Bob had. I met John when I went out dancing with a bunch of other Ricers. His interview took place in the parking lot of the Longbranch, a bar near Raleigh. John was from Great Neck, New York, and was single. He knew that his friend Bob had told me about his backslide, and he felt that he could provide an even cleverer tale of cheating. Some of the men I interviewed liked the one-upmanship of telling a better story. I enjoyed their competition because it was easier to interview them. They came to me instead of me having to track them down.

After two hours of the Watermelon Crawl and the Texas two-step, my heart rate reached its target range, and I signaled John to meet me outside. We squeezed into my cramped car and pushed the seats back as far as they could go. It was comical how small the car was and how large we were. We laughed to imagine how others saw us as they went in and out of the Longbranch. I balanced my notes on the steering wheel as John disconnected the shoulder harness. He smiled, pulled out a box of TicTacs, offered me one, and popped three in his mouth. He rolled them around and started talking.

John Frederick

"My first cheat was in Sin City. It is so close to the Rice House, you know they created it just for us. Even the new Rice House has a Sin City near it. I don't know what came first, the Rice House or Sin City, but since the Diet has been around since the 1930s, I guess the Diet was first and then the fast food joints found a captive market and built within walking distance of the Rice House. Just think, it's a can't-fail business arrangement. The Rice Diet packs in us fatsos to Durham, we are stuck here and starving, those restaurants spring up like mushrooms, and we indulge, gain weight, go back to the Rice House, starve, cheat, then back to the Rice House. It is the never-ending story.

"I never meant to go off the Diet. I swore to myself that I would not cheat. What was the point? I would be only cheating myself. I had been on program just a few weeks and was doing so well. Lost twenty-seven pounds and could even jog a couple of miles without straining. Everything was going great in my life. Then one night I just descended into food hell. I thought to myself that I deserved some kind of reward for staying on program, and it might as well be food. Yet this little voice inside my head said, 'No, no, don't do it.' I guess it was my good angel on my shoulder talking to me.

"I went to the weight room of my apartment building and worked out for about three hours, hoping that I could distract myself from the hunger. It didn't work. Finally I said, 'Fuck it. I am fat, I will always be fat, and who am I kidding?' Got in my car and headed straight for Sin City. Got to Dunkin' Donuts first and bought a dozen glazed and a dozen apple cinnamon, plus one large coffee with cream and Nutrasweet. I used Nutrasweet so I could pretend that I was still on a diet. In the parking lot I just devoured the donuts. Shoveled them in a handful at a time, like I couldn't get enough.

"Afterwards, I felt so high from all of that sugar that I just about passed out. I got into the back seat of my car and took a nap. I thought I was going to die, and they would find my car eventually. Realizing that there was a phone in my car, I called up a Ricer friend and told him the situation. I wanted him to do like an Overeaters Anonymous intervention and come rescue me from my despair. Instead, he said he would join me and to meet him at the Shoney's on Avondale Road. It was all-you-can-eat shrimp night.

"I met him there, and he brought along two old Ricers that I didn't know. Then all hell broke loose. We ate shrimp and French fries, drank real Cokes by the gallon and gobbled up two whole trays of hot fudge cakes. We ate and ate until the manager came over and said we couldn't eat any more shrimp because he had run out of it. I got mad because when a place says that they provide an all-you-can-eat buffet they should stand behind that.

"I didn't return to the Rice House for a week, and when I did everyone knew. Nobody said a word to me. They had all cheated too one time or another. The Rice House staff gave me a lecture, but hey, they aren't fat so they don't know what it's like."

John finished his story and looked at me, waiting for a response. He looked very proud of himself and his prodigious eating habits. I just sighed and shook my head, and he threw back his head and roared. I had to laugh too. His backslide was sad, even tragic, but funny too. John told me that he would see me at weigh-in in the morning. I watched as he waddled back into the building.

Jack Sizemore is a patron of Sin City also. I sought Jack out for an interview because he seemed the type who would never cheat. He was conscientious about the Diet, and I never knew him to be absent from the Rice House for any length of time. He didn't hang around with the known cheaters; he stuck pretty much to himself and occasionally would go out with others for coffee. I had never known him to miss a weigh-in. I knew Jack was married because I had met his wife and two children when they came to visit. Jack made them eat at the Rice House, so I knew he didn't use family as an excuse to eat off program.

I met Jack at the Mad Hatter, a little café and coffee bar not far from Duke's east campus and the Wall. I was there early and had time to check out the brightly lit cases of pastries and breads. There were rows of gigantic cookies with inch-high crowns of frosting. Rugalach as thick as bricks, and big, wide, open slices of cake almost obscene in their display. They showed all of their lovely, creamy layers to the attentive public. I was amazed at how erotic food could be. I thought of all this as I stood in line for my skim milk decaf tall latte. I glanced shyly at the slab of chocolate nut brownie staring at me. It did look good—rich, moist, dense, and black as night—but I knew I would be disappointed. I had been down that road before. It might have looked delicious, but it would not have been what I really wanted, which was the chocolate of my youth, the chocolate my mother used to make.

After the barista handed me my latte, I squeezed into a table and looked out the window for Jack. He was a half an hour late and very apologetic. He got himself a bottle of spring water and sat down. Jack looked good to me, healthy and tan, and I told him so. I wondered if he ever wanted to eat a chocolate brownie. He smiled, and I glanced down at my notes. I placed the tape recorder on the floor and draped the mike along the window ledge. Balancing my notebook on my lap, I asked Jack to start talking.

Jack Sizemore

"I feel rather stupid telling you this, but my first backslide was with a Meat Lovers pizza from Pizza Hut. This is a silly cheat for me because I could stay in New York and eat pizza, and the real thing too. I had been on program for four months, and I was getting buff. I was leaner than I had ever been in my life, and I worked out daily, ran six-mile sprints, and ate practically nothing, so I was really looking good. Hell, man, I thought I looked great. You could count my abs. I was down to about 172. Kempner's goal for me is 150 pounds, but I was looking good at 172.

"I was driving down the road after working out at MetroSport, and I saw that Pizza Hut marquee. It said they were having a two-for-one special on the Meat Lovers pizza. I pulled into the parking lot and went in. Nothing could stop me from having that pizza. I didn't even really want it, not the taste of it, but something inside of me just wanted to betray the Rice Diet. I sat down at the table and didn't even glance at the menu. I didn't need to because I knew what I wanted. I didn't even glance up at the waitress either. I ordered two extra-large hand-tossed Meat Lovers pizzas with extra cheese and two pitchers of beer. I had the waitress bring everything up on the table at once. I took such pleasure in just looking at all of the fat, greasy, salty food. I scarfed those pies down without actually tasting them and drained both pitchers. All I tasted was the salt and I knew my salt-deprived body was just soaking it up like a sponge. I didn't care. Nothing could stop me from that binge.

"When the waitress came back by I ordered another pizza to go: a Meat Lovers just like the other two. I paid my bill, took my pizza, and drove to the parking lot of Duke Towers. I sat in my car and slowly consumed the final pizza. Then I drove to Ken's Quik Mart and bought a pack of cigarettes and a six-pack of beer. I went back to my apartment and smoked one cigarette after another and drank the whole six-pack. I gained twenty-seven pounds in one night. My knees were so swollen that I couldn't stand up. I called up another Ricer, and he brought over some diuretics. I peed for three days, then walked in the Rice House as if nothing had happened."

Jack chuckled a little and shook his head. I couldn't believe he could backslide like that. I guess even the most dedicated dieter falls off the wagon now and then. I thanked him for the interview and watched him through the window as he walked to his car. I left a few moments later, but couldn't resist one last look at that brownie.

Some folks on the Diet consider themselves gourmets. They turn away from Sin City when they are heading for a binge, aiming instead for a better cheat. John Pettis is what I call a grand gourmet. His cheats were well known at the Rice House for their quality and style. If I hadn't known that John was a sixty-year-old physician, I would have thought that he was a young food critic for *Gourmet* or *Southern Living*. John looked ageless. His round face and body didn't provide any hints as to how old he was. He was also very interested in popular trends in music, literature, and art. He said his daughter and granddaughter kept him up to date. John was always tan and wearing white, as if he had just walked off of a tennis court. He was jolly and fun to be around, and he surrounded himself with several admiring women. I'd never seen John without a woman near him. He liked women, and they liked him. I enjoyed our interview and had my first (and last) cranberry martini at the bar in the Siena Hotel while I was taping John's story.

I walked into the lobby of the hotel to find John seated in the center of one of the plush sofas with a woman on either side of him. John didn't introduce me; instead he got up and took me by the arm to the bar. I looked back, and the women waved at me. John paid no attention to them. He ordered drinks for us and began talking. I whipped out my tape recorder, placed it on the bar, and punched the start button as fast as I could. There was no cassette in the recorder, and I had to fish one out of my bag. John began again.

John Pettis

"I have been to Durham several times now, and when I backslide it is not at some grease pit in Sin City. When I decide to cheat, I do so with a little style. People at the Rice House aren't your typical junk-food junkies anyway. We are used to fine dining and consider it a badge of honor that we have eaten at the best tables in the world. It is not as if we are snobs. Rather, we just know where to find good food. The food can be simple or sophisticated. Sin City does not have good food. The restaurants there merely stimulate the appetite, not satisfy it.

"The perfect backslide requires preparation. I must find the proper restaurant, the availability of a table, the wine cellar, and the selected company I will invite to my little feast. It takes me up to a week to prepare. I often go to the restaurant to review the menu and sample the wines. Sometimes I have an appetizer or two, but I don't consider that a true cheat, just a prelude. I go back to the Rice House and find some willing partners. That is not hard to do. The difficult part is to find the right companions.

"My favorite backslide is at the Fearrington House. It is the only five-star restaurant in the state of North Carolina, and they do a beautiful spread. If oysters are in season, I start out with some fresh, lightly battered ones on a bed of spinach leaves and a white wine. Then perhaps a soup, nothing with beans, preferably, but something light. The entrée can be anything, and I do take advice from the waiter. Usually it is something meat based and heavy, and I have a thick Merlot with it. I eat a few baskets of bread with butter too. Dessert is always chocolate mousse and coffee with Bailey's cream. If you eat like that, you don't need sex. I gain about five pounds per feast, but my lady friends are not that lucky. They gain around eight to ten pounds per cheat.

"The Rice House staff knows when I cheat, and they nag me about my blood pressure, my diabetes, and all the other diseases that I will get in the future, but for one lovely night I can transcend the monotony of that diet and just enjoy life."

He ordered another drink and wandered back to the lobby area. I didn't know if I should pay for my drink or let John pay for it. I tried to give the bartender five dollars, but he shooed me away. When I left the Siena, John was back on the sofa with the two women.

Henry Horace is also a grand gourmet. I met him for coffee at the Ninth Street Bakery for his interview. Like John Pettis, Henry was a ladies' man. I asked him what he did for a living and he said that he "financed things." He told me he had grown children as well as grown grandchildren and that his family members were scattered all over the world.

Despite his cheery nature, Henry often seemed sad to me. Even though he had many acquaintances at the Rice House and in Durham, I thought he was lonely. I knew he was ill because he would enter the hospital for a couple of weeks at a time and then show up at the Rice House. He never spoke of his illnesses, and I never asked him. I assumed they were the typical diseases of obesity and old age: heart disease and diabetes.

We sat near the door and drank one cup of coffee after another. He looked like he had done this many times before. I guess the monotony of the Diet was getting to him. He had been at the Rice House for years. Glancing out the window into the crowded parking lot, he started talking.

Henry Horace

"My biggest backslide event was at the Magnolia Grill. I decided if I was going to go to hell, I might as well do it with some style. I had heard about the Grill before I even came to Durham. I read about it in *Wine Spectator* magazine I think, and the article stuck in my mind. You know how it is when you are fat, you are always thinking about where to get that perfect meal. I had been on the Rice Diet for several months, and I had lost over a hundred pounds. I looked and felt like a new person.

"I had never eaten a meal outside of the Rice House. I had little cheats of course, a beer or two now and then and dry popcorn at the movies, but no big backslide. One day I decided to let it all go and just eat what I wanted. Funny because I had no great hunger; instead

I missed the flavor of food and how exquisite good food felt in my mouth and on my tongue. I missed alcohol too. I stopped drinking the night before I started the Rice Diet, and I missed it as much as the food. I decided that I would just enjoy myself like a normal person and have a night out. I asked a lovely lady that I had met on program to accompany me, and she said yes. I made reservations and called ahead and told the manager not to even bother to bring me a menu or wine list; I would leave the evening up to the staff.

"The meal was unbelievable. It took us four hours to eat it, and it cost three hundred dollars! It was worth every penny. I gained eight pounds in one night, and my date gained ten. I didn't cheat again until I was within ten pounds of goal weight, and then I went back to Magnolia Grill for one last fling in Durham."

Henry looked down into his coffee cup. He thought for a moment and drained it like shot a of whiskey. Then he slapped his hand on the table to signal the end of the interview and struggled to get up. I helped him get out of the chair and walk to his car. Henry looked embarrassed and grateful. Looking at him, I couldn't believe that he got so close to goal weight. No wonder he was sad. I went back inside and sat at our table watching people come and go for a hour or so, then drove home.

Brent Gruber is another grand gourmet. I also knew Brent in another context. He and I had worked for the same company several years before when I lived in Virginia. Brent was the second person I had met on the Rice Diet whom I had known previously. I thought this was very strange; perhaps there was an eating pattern peculiar to northern Virginia that made so many Ricers!

Brent owned a telecommunications company. He was fifty years old, married with four children, and lived in Vienna, Virginia. We used to stop at the coffee shop in the Pan Pan Diner after our walks. The diner looked like a Howard Johnson's motel, which it once had been; only the sign had been changed. The coffee was unbelievably bad and lukewarm, but the diner was about a mile and a half from the Rice House, so it was an easy walk after dinner.

Brent really liked to talk about eating and was often criticized by other Ricers for his preoccupation with food that was off limits.

One woman told me that she wouldn't even sit at a table with Brent because all of his talk about food made her nervous. Many people, including members of Overeaters Anonymous, believe that any reference to food should be forbidden. Even the naming of a particular food, such as chocolate or bread, can conjure up an unbearable hunger that might lead to a binge. This taboo may seem silly to a nondieter, but to those of us who have a deep, abiding love of food, the very naming of a certain food is reckless and can cause us to cheat.

Brent met me after his hike in Duke Forest. He was delighted that he was able to run the course without dying of a heart attack or a stroke. I drove him back to the Rice House, and we sat in the living room. No Ricers were around, just staff setting up for the next meal. Brent stretched out on a couch and flung his arms over his head. I sat in a chair and got out my trusty field notebook. We were in the classic patient and psychiatrist positions. Brent played along, folded his arms across his chest, and said, "Well, Doctor . . .

Brent Gruber

"My backslide was what I call a moveable feast. I gathered all of the food that I had missed on the Diet, had it prepared to my specifications, hauled it all to the Eno River, and had a pleasurable afternoon. I had made a list of all the food I loved and had to abandon forever. I did this the night before I started the Rice Diet. I kept the list and reviewed it from time to time, and I promised myself that when I had lost one hundred pounds, I would celebrate with a backslide to end all backslides. I know this seems so illogical to thin people, but fat people understand. There is this huge longing for food; it's not even the taste so much as the promise of it. I just can't let go of the food, and I don't think any other fat person can either, no matter what they say or how thin they get. The food is always waiting.

"When I lost my hundred pounds, I got into my car and drove straight to Foster's Gourmet Market to start things going. Then I went to A Southern Season, and finally to that restaurant in the Siena Hotel. I got thick, crusty loaves of bread, a variety of salads, including fried chicken salad, all types of cheeses—especially the semi-soft ones, you know, the ones that are always off-limits to dieters—I just bought everything I desired. I went to the Siena and convinced the chef to prepare me some veal piccata and pasta for take-out. I loaded all of those delicious, forbidden, delightful selections in the back of my SUV and went to the Eno River. A few other Ricers showed up and some had brought dessert! We all cheated. The four of us sat on the banks of the Eno, ate and drank like old times, smoked a couple of joints, and just enjoyed life again. I knew that the backslide would cause me pain in the future, and I would have to stay in Durham longer and eat even more rice and fruit, but that one glorious afternoon was worth it."

Brent patted his little potbelly and grinned like the Cheshire Cat, delighted both with his feast and the telling of it. He hopped up and looked expectantly at me, waiting for a reaction. I applauded dutifully and told him his was the best backsliding story I had heard. He looked pleased as he walked toward the dining room for lunch. I followed him to a table and, over a bowl of rice, thought about his lovely picnic on the Eno.

Nathan Patel left the country to have his backsliding event. I knew Nathan from the tales of derring-do and sexual conquests that littered his dinner-table conversations. He kidded everyone, and there was an underlying sexual tone in everything he said. He was crude and even ridiculous. I didn't want to interview him, but after I heard of his backsliding tale, I approached him for an interview, and he agreed. We arranged to meet in a very public place. I didn't want to be alone with him because he was sort of creepy.

We met at Northgate Mall. Nathan and I got a couple of cups of coffee and found an available table. The food court was crowded, noisy, and bright. Looking around at the people, the food vendors, and the screaming children, I felt a headache coming on. I was keeping tabs on a group of Ricers I spied checking out the free samples at the Mrs. Fields cookie counter. The women were taking little samples of the cookies. Nathan glanced around to see what I was watching and laughed. I didn't know if I would even be able to record his words in this environment, but thought I would give it a try. I turned up the volume on the tape recorder as high as possible and wasn't paying much attention to Nathan as he began his tale.

Nathan Patel

"I have the grandest backsliding story of all. I had been on the Rice Diet six months, and I lost 127 pounds. I was in remarkable shape and off all medication. I was feeling good and looking good. Then one day I just decided that I didn't want to do it anymore, didn't want to be on a diet. I knew that I had to lose more weight, and I had to diet to do that, but I just didn't want to. I decided to cheat a little and then get back in the swing of things. I decided that I would take a week and do what I wanted, to see how I would do when I was back out in the real world of food. I promised myself that I could have anything in the world I wanted.

"What I wanted was a club sandwich from this hotel in London that I had stayed in once. So I flew to London. I flew four other Ricers with me, and we had a ball. We were like inmates escaped from prison. We stayed at the Dorchester. We ate and drank the whole time. I know I must have slept, but all I remember is the eating and drinking. When we showed up again at the Rice House the staff was very upset with us, but some of the Ricers stood up and applauded."

Nathan spoke of his adventure as an everyday occurrence, as if anybody could fly to London for a sandwich. I was amazed. He assured me that it wasn't the first time he had flown somewhere for a meal, but it was the first time he'd backslid on the Rice Diet. I didn't think it odd that someone could want a sandwich or a particular type of food so much that they would leave the country for it. I could probably name every meal I ever had, especially the best one—which was in Sweden, of all places. I bet everyone at the Rice House could tell you where to find the best pizza, the greatest cinnamon bun, or the perfect apple pie. What got me was the idea of having enough disposable money to act on these desires. I was impressed. As I left the food court, I looked around for the Ricers at the cookie counter. They had worked their way around to TCBY and were gobbling up little bites of yogurt. They probably didn't even think they were cheating. The samples at the food court may be small and free, but they cost you at the scale. They would learn. Nathan and I decided to walk back to the Rice House. We would pick up our cars later.

I liked the way men backslide. They do it with such decisiveness and flair. We women don't engage in a grand backslide. Instead, our little cheats on the Diet are the sins of opportunity. We don't plan to eat off the Diet. We don't fly to London or create a moveable feast. We don't fall off the wagon but rather slide off. Our cheats are random.

Barbara Hirshfeld considers herself a typical Ricer. She doesn't cheat so much as slide off the Diet. I met her at one of her favorite places to slip into a backslide, A Southern Season. I was late for our meeting, and when I found Barbara she was already laying into a portobello mushroom sandwich. She was on what she called a dieting holiday. Although she was cheating on the Diet, she didn't see it that way because she wasn't officially dieting.

I didn't know Barbara well. She came and went at the Rice House like so many others. I didn't get close to her because she came with her own crew—fellow dieters who spent a little time in Durham on the way to someplace else, usually Florida. She was always well-groomed, and I felt conspicuous around her because what I wore seemed thrown together.

For the interview she showed up as her usual spectacular self. Her blonde hair was stylishly cut and swung when she turned her head. Her pantsuit was tailor made and accentuated her large but well-shaped body. My hair was sticking out, my socks were falling down, my pants were too baggy, and my old sweater was stretched out. I felt like a blob next to Barbara.

As I slid into the booth, Barbara reluctantly put down her sandwich. You could tell she was really enjoying her dieting holiday. She dabbed the corners of her mouth without disturbing her lipstick and began explaining herself.

Barbara Hirshfeld

"I never really had a big backslide like some people I know. I realize this is a difficult diet, but the only way to get through it is to just follow it. If you screw around too much you get lost. I have had legal cheats—not legal to the Rice House, but legal to any other diet. I don't set out to cheat, but things just happen.

"I was here at A Southern Season one day to get some good coffee. That is what I miss most when I am on program—a good cup of coffee. That Sanka they give you at the Rice House is terrible. A Southern Season has free little cups of good coffee with real cream and brown sugar granules. I started out with a couple of those, and God did they taste like heaven. Then I had a free sample of the chocolates at the candy counter. Before I knew it I had worked my way around the entire store. I was sampling this and tasting that: chocolate, cheese, bread, cookies, salami, and even a thimbleful of wine. I don't know how it happened. I just intended to have a coffee. I just couldn't stop myself.

"I put on three pounds with those little samples. I told Dr. Kempner that I gained weight because I had my period. I don't think he believed me, or that he even cared, but I had to say something. I felt like a fool. I try to stay away from those places, but every now and then I just end up somewhere that has free food, and that's all it takes for me to cheat.

"Sometimes a few of my friends will get together, and it just happens: we go off the Diet a little bit. We don't intend to cheat, we don't have any intentions whatsoever, we just run into food everywhere. I guess you could say we are food junkies looking for a fix and if one of us cheats, then we all do. We influence each other's behavior. I know that I have the strength to say no, but when I am with a group of others who are eating off program, I just go along with the flow."

Barbara finished half her sandwich and pushed the other half away. She was showing great willpower. We both got up, and I paid the bill and headed for the door. Barbara wanted to take one last look around the store and headed to the candy counter.

When I got to know Barbara better, she and her friends took me shopping. I got the cheapest and best-fitting black crepe jacket in the world with a matching skirt on that spree, and I still have it today. When Barbara or one of her friends lost weight, they would drop their old clothes off at my house. Soon I had turned in my old grad-student clothes and was wearing couture. I felt like Cinderella at the ball. After I had known Barbara for six months she took me to her stylist and had my hair cut short and close to my head. I think of Barbara every time I need a haircut.

Alexa Dellon, a twenty-one-year-old student originally from California, cheats but tries to stay within the frame of healthy eating. I met her at the location of her original backslide, the China Inn in Durham. The staff there is used to dieters and has a special section on their menu devoted to entrees that are low in fat, calories, and sodium. Alexa and I shared an dish of steamed vegetables and white rice prepared without salt or flavorings of any kind. Alexa ate a forkful of broccoli and took a sip of tea. She put down her cup and stared at it for a few moments and then started talking.

Alexa Dellon

"About three months into the program, I just had this overwhelming urge to eat something crunchy and good. I was sick and tired of rice and fruit. I couldn't gag down another spoonful of that slop they give you at the Rice House, and I was determined that I would have something decent. I didn't want to totally blow all of the progress I had made, I didn't want to gain much weight, but I was willing to put on a pound or two for the taste of something good. I decided that I could get away with some Chinese food if I stuck to selections that were not battered and fried and not loaded with sauce, MSG, or sodium.

"I chose the China Inn as my place to backslide because I had heard from Ricers that you could get a good meal Ricer-style, without sugar or salt. I checked out the parking lot to make sure no Ricers and especially no Rice House staff were around. I went up to the carry-out area and placed my order. I had decided on a stir-fry composed of chicken and a ton of vegetables, along with steamed rice. Okay, I added an egg roll or two, but that was it. I was sitting at the bar waiting for my order, when out of the corner of my eye I saw Dr. Newborg and some of the staff from the Rice House! I could not believe it. Before they could see me I slithered off the stool and darted to the kitchen. I figured the kitchen would have a back door and I could make my escape without any of the Rice House staff seeing me.

"The kitchen itself was a madhouse. Everyone was screaming in Chinese, and there were piles and piles of raw meat. People were chopping away with cleavers. Some man came up to me and started yelling in Chinese, and I couldn't understand one word, but I got the drift. I shouted back that I had to go in secrecy, that I couldn't leave by the main entrance because I didn't want to be seen by certain people in the dining room. He seemed to understand this and looked relieved. He showed me to the back door and I started to leave, and then I said, 'I need my food.' I was not going to leave without the food!

"He grabbed one of the white bags that were piled up in the kitchen and shut the door in my face. I slunk to my car, got in, and drove back to my apartment. When I got home I looked in the bag, and to my delight there was a big box full of General Tso's chicken, fried wontons, sweet and sour soup with those crunchy fried noodles, and a small container of white rice. I thought that God himself had decided that I should have a decent meal as a reward for all of my suffering on the Rice Diet. I ate all of it so fast I didn't have time to even think about the consequences. Something just came over me, and I ate and ate. I gained seven pounds and was sick for a couple of days, but I will never forget how good that meal tasted."

Alexa smiled and sat back. She was convinced that fate, rather than her actions, had caused the backslide. The Lord does work in mysterious ways. I wondered when the Lord would act again and Alexa would backslide. We agreed that there was no understanding the will of God. I left her there to ponder these things as I paid the bill. She waved as I walked out the door.

Angelina Sarafina got caught on her first backslide in Durham.

She was a reporter from Dallas, Texas, and very new to diet culture. She had recently married, and, to her surprise, she put on a lot of weight very quickly. Because her job was at stake due to her weight gain, she and her television station chose the Rice Diet as a fast way to lose weight. I met her and her husband at the Rice House, and she volunteered her backslide story at our first meeting. She and her husband now thought it funny, but hadn't thought so when it occurred a few weeks earlier.

I met with Angelina on the Rice House porch. She was very beautiful and looked like the Madonna from a Renaissance painting. Her body was big but compact, and her dark face was perfectly shaped. She wore her long hair in a braid down her back. She looked about sixteen, but I knew she was probably in her early thirties. When she laughed, she covered her mouth with her hands. As I set up the tape recorder, Angelina asked me to hurry. She didn't want to be late to a step aerobics class. I snapped a cassette in place and told her to start talking.

Angelina Sarafina

"I got caught cheating on my very first backslide. Such bad luck! I was so good on the Rice Diet, a saint of the program. Dr. Newborg used to parade me out in front of all the new recruits and tell them how good I was, how much weight I had lost, and how honest I was to the Diet. I was so proud and I guess a bit of a snob because I used to look down my nose at those people who ate off program. How could they do it? I thought they were very common, very low people to disregard the Diet so. The Diet was what was saving us and here were people who were just flaunting their bad behavior. I didn't associate with any of them or sit at their table. Everyone knew they were cheaters. I never thought it would be me, but one night, the seventh of June at 6:34 p.m., I decided I had to have some chocolate. I remember the precise time because I was driving when the urgency hit me. I know the date because it was the day my husband was coming to visit me. I was to pick him up at nine that evening.

"I wanted a few chocolates, that was all. I wanted the kind you get from a real candy counter, the kind they put in a white paper bag. The only place in Durham I knew of that had these chocolates was Fowler's in Brightleaf Square, and I knew they closed at seven p.m. I drove down the road, whirled into the parking lot, and ran into the store. It is not as though I actually planned to backslide. When I got in my car I wasn't intending to go to Fowler's; it was as though the car had a preset destination.

"The girl behind the counter in the store was in a hurry and wanted me to make a selection quickly because they were closing. I wanted to take my time because I wanted the backslide to be precisely what I needed—not just any old chocolate, but something worthy of the event. This sin was a big deal to me, and I knew it would cost me, but I knew I would commit it, I would indulge. I selected four pieces of Neuhaus solid chocolates, two English toffees, and four dark chocolate bonbons with white cream filling. To make it an even twelve I told the girl to toss in a couple for luck. She probably thought I was nuts, but she did it anyway and said nothing. She put all of them in a white paper bag, the proper way.

"I strolled quickly to my car because I didn't want anyone from the Rice House to see me. All of Durham is crawling with Ricers and staff. I made it safely to my car. I drove to the parking lot of Duke Chapel, rolled down the windows, and took the first bite from the Neuhaus solid. I let it linger on my tongue until the chocolate was totally melted. I continued this process for the next two pieces, but then alternated between hard bites and the slow and melting ones. Sometimes, I would just suck the chocolate through my teeth.

"I had no idea what time it was, and when I turned on the car, I saw that it was almost nine, and I still had to drive to Raleigh to meet my husband's plane. I stuffed those little candy ruffled brown paper things in the white bag and jammed it up under the car radio. It was the first place I thought of. I drove to the airport and met my husband's plane on time.

"He was so delighted by the way I was beginning to look and was sort of stunned by my weight loss. I was nervous about seeing him. I wanted him to be proud of me, and he told me he was. He said he was proud of my weight loss and of the time and dedication I put into taking the weight off. He also missed me and was anxious for me to get to my goal weight so I could come home to him. We had only been married four months when I started the Diet. We were still on a honeymoon.

"On the way home, a policeman pulled me over and said I had a taillight that was out. Okay, no big deal. Then for some reason—I assume it was because we are not Anglo—he decided to search the car. He asked us to get out of the car and then he shined the flashlight all around. Then he reached up under the dashboard and started searching around. He found that white paper bag and pulled it out. When he did, all of those brown paper wrappers fluttered out across the floor of the car. The police officer and my husband stared at me, and I just shrugged. My husband did not say one word to me the rest of the evening."

Angelina got up and gathered up her equipment for her aerobics class. She seemed a little embarrassed by her backslide. I thought it hysterically funny and told her so. She shrugged her shoulders and waved me off. I watched as she bounded down the stairs to the parking lot, curious to know if there was any candy in her glove compartment.

Harriet Wolk's backslide landed her in the hospital. Harriet was from Portland, Oregon and had her own television program. She was a painter and the editor of an arts magazine. Harriet was married with one son. She reminded me of every grade school teacher I ever had. You know the type: someone who is kind and gentle and wears denim jumpers and sensible flat shoes straight out of an L. L. Bean catalog. Harriet carried a tote bag she had made from quilt patches and was wearing handmade dangling silver earrings. She didn't swear and would look worried when others did. I liked Harriet. During the interview, I was astounded to find that she had cheated on her husband as well as the Diet.

We met at my house for the interview, and I served water. Harriet wouldn't drink tea, not even herbal, because she felt it stimulated appetite. She got out her knitting from one of the bags she always carried and began her work. I set up and told her to begin talking. Without looking up or missing a stitch, she started to speak.

Harriet Wolk

"My backslide was at the San Francisco International Airport. One must be totally desperate to eat airport food, but there are some decent places in the airport, and besides, after rice and fruit for three months anything tastes divine. I was going to meet an old lover—not my husband—at the airport, and we were going to drive down the coast to Carmel for a weekend. We have a same-time-next-year type of relationship, and I looked forward to our yearly lovefest.

"My plane got in early, so I decided to have a cheat. Who would know? I was clear across the country from the Rice House, and nobody knew me in San Francisco. I went to this snack bar and ordered two cheeseburgers on sourdough buns, a double order of French fries, the kind with the skins still on them, and two Bass Ales. I ate and drank until that calmness you get from food came over me. I looked up at the monitor and saw that my friend's plane had come in, but it didn't really register. After a while, I heard my name being called over the intercom. I picked up the courtesy phone, and it was my friend asking where I was. While I was waiting for him, I had another beer and a order of those fried cheese sticks. He met me and we drove down to Carmel.

"I started to feel ill on the way down, but I assumed it was merely a bad case of car sickness. Later on that night, I thought that I might be having one of those horrible reactions to forbidden food that you hear about in Ricer fables. By midnight I was in the emergency room with a hot appendix. The ER doctor asked me the name and address of my family physician, and I blurted out 'Rice House.' When I got back to the Rice House, Dr. Kempner just shook his head in disgust. I never saw my boyfriend again."

Harriet looked up at me over her little reading glasses to register my response. I was truly flabbergasted. Imagining her as a sex siren cavorting with lovers in secret hideaways was beyond me. I didn't know what to say. Harriet smiled, satisfied that she had shocked me. She asked if she could stay a while and watch a soap opera. We watched three hours of afternoon television shows, the characters jumping in and out of bed with everyone except their spouses. Around four o'clock she gathered her things and left. I saw her an hour later at the Rice House. She was still knitting.

Susan Littleton's backslide also put her in the hospital. Susan described herself as a middle-aged wife and mother from Atlanta, Georgia, as well as a former runner-up in the Miss America contest. She was the CEO of a major food company. Susan was Southern, short, and bouncy, with big hair. She had an open, go-getting personality and always looked on the sunny side of things. I didn't like her at first because she reminded me of an over-the-hill cheerleader or an overactive Girl Scout. I could just picture Susan leading a bunch of girls on an overnight camping trip. Still, I interviewed her because she had a good story. Later I learned to like her, and we went to the movies a couple of times. Her good cheer wore down my reluctance to be her friend. I still get a Christmas card from her every year and a Holly Farms box of sausage rolls and cheese sticks.

We met at the Rice House before dinner. The place was practically empty. We sat in the living room and Susan leafed through some old magazines someone had left on the coffee table. Every few moments she would absentmindedly touch her hair to make sure it was still in place. I didn't think anything could disturb that hair. I wondered if it was a wig. I asked her to just start talking about backslides. She put down the magazine, crossed her ankles, looked down at her French-manicured nails, and started talking.

Susan Littleton

"My first backslide ended with a stay in the emergency room at Duke. I was doing so well on the Rice Diet and felt absolutely gorgeous. I felt young and pretty and single. I was deeply in love. I felt powerful and courageous and had all of this self-confidence because I was doing so well on the Diet. I was almost to goal weight. Everyone knew that I would reach it within three weeks, four at the most. I was thin and looking good. I had never, never cheated on the Diet. What would be the point? I was in Durham to diet and to get back in shape so my old friends would speak to me again. Everyone at the Rice House was so proud of me. They would show my before picture at morning rounds, and then point to me and say, 'We are so proud, Susan.' I felt like the chosen one. I was the one who would do it: reach goal weight, keep off the weight, and live thin happily ever after.

"One Friday night, I was out with my boyfriend and we were going to go to Squid's for a quick drink. Actually, he was going to drink, I was going to watch. I usually have a seltzer with lime, but this time I wanted something more. I decided to have one glass of Chardonnay. One tiny glass, 120 calories, no sodium. I didn't think I would gain any weight with that one glass. Squid's was having a two-for-one special on oysters. I love raw oysters with Texas Pete hot sauce. We ordered some, and then more and more, and the shells kept piling up at the bar in front of us. I had that little knife they give you to pry open the oysters and on the thirteenth oyster, I slipped and ran the knife clean through the palm of my left hand. Blood squirted all over the bar and the bartender called 911 and gave me a towel. The EMS people insisted I go to Duke to have them look at my hand. I didn't want to go because I felt like such a fool and so guilty.

"At Duke it took eight stitches to sew up my hand, and when I showed up at the Rice House the next morning everyone knew. I shouldn't have had that last oyster. The thirteenth one was my downfall."

Susan finished her story and jumped up to run around the Rice House a few times. She didn't like to sit in one position very long and insisted that sitting for a length of time would lower metabolism and increase the likelihood of weight gain. Also, she informed me that sitting caused varicose and spider veins. I shuddered and felt my legs tingle. When I left the Rice House, Susan was doing a set of deep-knee squats. Never say die, I thought to myself as I left the parking lot.

I never backslid in Durham. I stayed on rice and fruit for four months and didn't even drink a glass of water that was not from the Rice House. My cheat was in Florida, where I went to the home of a fellow Ricer for the Christmas holidays. My first backslide was with a common hot dog—not even a great hot dog, but the kind they serve in airports and bars. I ate it at the snack bar at a golf course. I gained five pounds.

Backsliding is something most of us do. When we begin the Diet, we find the idea of cheating incredible. We've spent all of this time and money and effort just to get to Durham; why would we destroy everything for some temporary pleasure, a few morsels of food? Yet time and again the power of food conquers us and we give in. The men among us cheat in a grand way; the women have their secret meetings with food.

For many of us, cheating is the ultimate but requisite sin that moves us to a deeper understanding of dieting. We attack the Diet with a new fervor and view dieting as a religious quest. We become Diet worshippers.

nine

Diet Worship

All of us take the requirements of the Diet to heart. That's how we lose weight. But to most of us, the Rice Diet is just a diet, and eventually we will go off it. We've been on hundreds of diets, succeeded on most of them, went off all of them, and gained back the weight. The Rice Diet is no different in this respect. We lose weight in Durham, then go home and gain most, if not all, of it back. Yet there are those in diet culture who succeed in incorporating the essence of the Rice Diet into their very souls. They view it as a way of life and a code for proper behavior, much like the Bible or the Koran. To them the world is divided into what is acceptable and what is taboo. Pure food is anything that is served in the Rice House; food that is off limits is anything available outside the Rice House and is part of the fallen world. People who practice good dieting skills are viewed as saints; cheaters are seen as sinners. The hierarchical god of the Rice Diet is the late Dr. Kempner. To Diet worshippers he is the founder and spiritual leader of Diet culture, and his teachings and proverbs still form, inspire, and instruct his followers. Dieters who practice their faith in the Rice Diet lose more weight and keep it off longer than the rest of us. They don't view it as a diet but as a prescription for health, happiness, and spiritual healing. They don't go on and off the Diet; they live it every day of their lives.

The transformation of self is very difficult. Religious ethos provides an image of the ideal transformation. Dieters in the process of losing weight view themselves as noble, courageous, and up to the struggle with unforeseen obstacles as well as with daily and familiar temptations of the flesh. Worshippers repeat tales of saints who have resisted the urges of appetites and passed by the all-you-can-eat buffets that make up Durham. They tell of miracles where people were actually cured of their obesity and never again experienced a night of bingeing followed by a morning of purging. They seek ritual atonement and sacred, magical foods with negative calories, such as grapefruit and rice. To them, the struggle for weight loss is more about character and personal discipline than about poundage lost. Women more than men see dieting as a religion, and this view addresses the core experience of dieting women in Western culture. To us, dieting is a moral as well as physical quest.

I met Linda Catesano the first week I was on the Rice Diet. She helped me survive the first few days on program. She had been on the Diet for a long time and knew a lot about diet culture. When I had a question, I asked Linda, not the doctors of the Rice House. I figured Linda was an authority on losing weight because she had lost a lot of it, and the others on the Diet looked to her for inspiration. She was always encouraging and believed everyone could lose weight if they followed the Diet.

Linda was married and had a toddler at home in Toms River, New Jersey. At the time, I was shocked that she could leave a husband and child for such a long period, but Linda told me she had no choice. No diet program worked for her except the Rice Diet. She wasn't very large when I met her, but she had lost over a 150 pounds at the Rice House. She went home a couple of weeks later and didn't return for months. When she came back, it was because she had regained half her weight and was determined to stay until she reached goal, no matter how long it took. With that in mind, Linda moved to Durham permanently. She was still married, and her husband and child visited her a couple of times a month. Her husband was trying to get a job in Durham so his family could live together.

I met with Linda in her townhouse. I was surprised that she didn't live closer to the Rice House: wouldn't it be easier to walk to the Rice House rather than drive? Later, I found out from other Ricers that Linda did walk to the Rice House—a seven-mile trek each way.

Linda was waiting for me on the steps as I pulled into the parking lot. She showed me into her house and gave me a tour. There were a couple of pieces of furniture in each room, but that was all. No television, no piles of books and magazines, not even any newspapers. The kitchen was spotless, and I didn't see any small appliances, equipment, utensils, or plates. Stuck with a pig magnet to the refrigerator door was what I assumed to be Linda's before picture. The photo was of a huge blob of a human being dressed in black. I guessed it to be a female, but I couldn't be sure. The hair was very short and the features distorted. The whole aspect of it was that of some medical mishap. Linda saw me gaping at it, and when I turned, she nodded to me. It *was* her! It was hard to believe that the thin woman standing next to me was the same one as the freak on the refrigerator. As I stood there, not knowing what to say, I realized what I must have looked like to others before my weight loss. Linda read my thoughts and took me by the hand, away from the horrific photo and up the stairs to the second floor.

The bedroom had a single bed shoved against the wall. On the nightstand was a phone, a Bible, and a photograph of her husband and child. Running shoes, jump rope, and two pink hand weights were neatly stacked against a closet door. I took a seat on the floor and plugged my tape recorder into the nearest outlet. Linda sat on the floor opposite me and folded her long tanned legs under her into a meditation position. She placed each hand on her knees, palms up, and centered herself. She looked down at her sternum as she started talking.

Linda Catesano

"The first time I was at the Rice House I didn't know what was really going on. I was just out of college and went to Durham to lose about a hundred pounds. Once I got there though, I just partied the whole time and didn't lose all of my weight. I lost fifty pounds, went home and gained it all back in two months. Of course, everyone back home thought I was a winner because I'd lost fifty pounds, but I knew it wasn't true. That is how the world is; it even praises your failures. Dr. Kempner would have said I was a failure because I was still overweight, and he would have been right. Back home I felt pretty good about the weight I had lost, but in my heart I knew it wasn't enough. You could ask a hundred people, and they would tell you the same story. I just didn't get the concept of the Rice Diet the first time I was in Durham. I thought a diet was something you went on, then went off once you lost your weight. You see, I was still in love with food and with my old lifestyle. I didn't know that dieting required a change in heart as well as in behavior.

"The second time the Rice Diet took root in me, and I began to understand that obesity is a spiritual as well as physical disease. I had this big empty hole inside me that I was trying to fill all the time but couldn't fill completely. I tried food, sex, drugs, exercise, even God, but nothing worked. The Rice Diet does. It soothes the storm in my soul and takes away my huge longing for food. I feel so peaceful on rice and fruit, and almost ethereal.

"I became a Christian because of the Rice Diet. I converted to Catholicism at that little chapel on the campus of North Carolina Central University. I went there every morning when I began the Diet and begged God to change me. I was raised without any religious orientation to speak of. I was born a Jew, but my parents were pretty much nonpracticing. My grandmother was another story. She kept kosher, but my mom wasn't into all of that. My mother thinks religion is a waste of time. I never went to temple or even thought about religion except on the high holidays. God just wasn't central to my life. I believed in a sort of vague higher power. Not a power directly involved in my everyday life and problems, but a distant one who sat up high somewhere and spun the world around. God didn't have any influence on me, and I had no influence on God—until the Rice Diet. I was born again at the Rice House. I got a new body thanks to the Diet, but also a new soul.

"My family and old friends have nothing much to do with me. Some of them think I am a religious zealot because of my eating and exercise habits. I am very faithful to my regimens. They aren't *my* regimens, but those of Dr. Kempner. Remember when he used to tell us that the only way to keep the weight off was to remind ourselves each day that we are different from other people and must make dieting our number one priority? It is the absolute truth. If you don't put the Diet ahead of everything else in your life, you will gain back the weight and live in regret forever.

"I know this is hard for the majority of people to do. After all, we live in the world, and the world is full of eating events, temptations of high-fat, high-calorie, and high-sodium food. We can always find some excuse not to exercise. We can also find some reason to excuse our fat. We convince ourselves that it is our metabolism, lifestyle, or situation when what we are really saying is that we don't have the guts or discipline to lose weight. It is hard to lose weight and keep it off, but it can be done. I am a walking testament to that.

"I have a very spartan lifestyle compared to the rest of America. I rent an apartment that I call minimalist. I don't have a lot of furniture or adornments in the place because they are unnecessary and just clutter up my life with stuff. I go to mass as often as possible because it is the way I renew myself. I like to go as early in the morning as I can to get the day started off right. Then I come home and have breakfast, which is one cup of cereal and one fruit. I keep a measuring cup right next to the cereal box so I can't cheat. I eat exactly eight ounces of high-fiber cereal or plain oatmeal and one small orange. For lunch I have a cup of rice and two fruits, usually peaches and grapes. Dinner is another cup of rice and two more fruits. Sometimes, for variety's sake, I will exchange the rice for some spoon-size shredded wheat, just like we ate at the Rice House. Twenty-two shredded wheat bites equal a rice exchange. It goes without saying that I don't eat any dairy, meat, sugar, or salt.

"I do fourteen miles of power walking a day. It takes me forever to do it, and I try to get it out of the way as soon as possible. Three times a week I work out with weights at the YMCA, and on Tuesdays and Thursdays I do abdominal work to tighten my stomach muscles. I think I will have to get plastic surgery to remove my apron and generally re-drape all of my loose skin.

"I am faithful to the Rice Diet as put forth by Dr. Kempner. He knew what he was doing. The inheritors of the Rice House are in no way as inspiring as Dr. Kempner, but they do follow most of his Diet even though they have changed things. The Rice Diet will continue no matter who runs it.

"Some people view me as an example of the Diet, as some sort of saint. I know that they show my picture around, and my name is still up on the Century Board at the Rice House. I have managed to maintain my goal weight, but I am in no way a saint. I struggle every hour with compliance, because my body wants to run out and eat as much food as possible, and of the most destructive kind. I long for something fat and greasy. My heart, however, prefers the pureness of the Diet. Sometimes when I am just so stressed out that I can't hear my heart and my body is demanding dangerous food, I just remember what Dr. Kempner said, 'Do it, do it, do it.' Do the Rice Diet; don't think about it. When everything else fails, rely on the Diet to take hold. That's what I do."

Linda finished her story and stretched out her legs. Absentmindedly, she bent her forehead to one of her knees and quietly counted to ten. In one swift movement, she got up from the floor and smiled down at me. Looking at her, it was impossible to believe that she had at one time been that sad person pictured on the door of her empty refrigerator. I uncrossed my stiff, bulky legs and doubted that I would get up with any kind of style. I wasn't thin and graceful like Linda, but I was strong: with a lunge, I hurled myself up from the floor. Linda looked pleased and walked me down to the front door. When I left, she was putting on her ankle weights and heading out for a run.

I got into my Tercel and said a silent prayer of thanks for people like Linda, who were inspirations to people like me. As I turned on the ignition and backed out of the parking lot, I also thanked God for Manchester, England, home of the Industrial Revolution. I thanked Him for the combustible engine, and Henry Ford, and all of those people and events who brought forth the car I was driving in, thus saving me from walking the seven miles back to the Rice House.

I met Karen Blackwell at Duke Chapel. I had seen her off and on at Ricer haunts and sometimes at the Rice House. Karen wasn't actually on program any more, but she did visit now and then to check in and to size up the new recruits. Karen used to give me the creeps. She was someone who was quite critical in her appraisals of a dieter's potential weight loss. I didn't like her. Still, she was someone to contend with and someone who knew everything there was to know about diet culture. She traded gossip. You would tell Karen something and she would tell you a little more about that person. Some referred to her as the town crier. Many were afraid to say anything of value in front of her.

What I knew about Karen's personal life I found out through gossip. I couldn't confirm the truth of it because Karen refused to reveal any part of her past. Karen was approximately sixty-five years old and a retired federal worker from Silver Spring, Maryland. She had been a follower of the Rice Diet since around 1988. She was divorced and had grown children and grandchildren.

I wanted to interview her because she was seen as an elder of the Rice Diet and someone to whom I should pay my respects. She agreed to talk to me about the Diet, but would not answer any questions. She would speak and I would listen.

I was surprised when Karen asked if we could meet at her place. It was rumored that no one was allowed there. As I drove down the highway to the apartment complex, I tried to picture what her apartment would look like. Surely it would be a dark place, something like a cave. When Karen opened her door and invited me in, I realized that I wasn't too far off the mark. The apartment was dark and cramped. Although the day was sunny, Karen had drawn the heavy brown draperies, and I immediately felt claustrophobic. I sat down on the dark brown sofa, and Karen sat on a chair opposite me. She didn't ask if I wanted anything to eat or drink, and I got out my stuff. Looking around at the depressing room, I asked if we could open the sliding glass doors to get in a little fresh air. Karen blinked a couple of times, but did as I requested. As I pulled out my notebook, she began her testimony.

Karen Blackwell

"I don't believe in God like a lot of worshippers do. I mean, what is the point? Look at the world. If there was a God, there's no way He would allow so many horrible things to happen. I don't believe in religion of any sort. I don't like all of that mumbo jumbo. I mean, what is all this sacrifice on the cross and blood of a lamb and water to wine? I don't believe it. But the Rice Diet I do believe. Ask and ye shall receive. I wanted to get thin, and I got thin. Amen and Hallelujah. Thank God. Thank Kempner. I believe in the Rice Diet. I believe in the rules of it. You do right, don't sin, and you get that pie in the sky: goal weight. You screw up, you gain weight, descend into fat hell, and it serves you right. You pay for your sins. Fat people like us unfortunately wear our sins. Hell is when you are at your fattest. I believe in purgatory too. Purgatory to me is when you have lost weight but not enough weight, and you can't get motivated to lose more. You are in suspended animation. Your weight just snowballs, and you go spiraling from one diet program to another.

"I guess some people could call the Rice Diet a religion. Dr. Kempner was our high priest, or rabbi. Our confessional is our weigh-in, and the rice and fruit is the food of the faithful—manna for the people struggling to get to the promised land. I guess the Rice House itself is our church. The Rice Diet is the only religion that I know of that truly delivers. You don't have to wait until you are dead to get your just reward, you just follow the path that others have gone, and you get thin."

Karen got up, slammed the balcony door, and jerked the curtains shut. That was it; the interview was over. She showed me to the door. I didn't see her again for weeks, and when I did, we didn't speak but merely nodded to each other in passing.

I interviewed Annie Jenkins at the Eno River in Durham. Annie agreed to an interview if I would not interrupt her exercise schedule. She would give me her story as we hiked a trail. She was very athletic, and I could barely believe that she had ever been really fat. She looked so tan and blonde that I just assumed that she had been a professional tennis or golf player. I knew that she had once been married to the CEO of a financial investment firm, but they were now separated. She had one grown daughter, and a teenage son.

I liked Annie because she was free. She was totally focused on living an authentic life, and for her that meant a life devoted to thinness. She was very disciplined, but did not look down on those like me who were not.

Keeping up with Annie was rough. We didn't jog but walked swiftly over the trail near the river. I had my tape recorder plastered to my back, and I held the microphone up and away from me. I was hoping that it would pick up Annie's words instead of my strained breathing. I watched Annie as she walked up the path in front of me. Her hair streamed down her back, and her arms pumped up and down like she was leading a marching band. The backs of her sinewy calves had hard little balls on them. Her thighs bulged with muscles and were the biggest part of her. I felt sweat trickle down between my breasts and was relieved to see sweat starting to form on Annie's back. I wasn't the only one feeling the hike. My shins began to ache, and I asked if we could stop now. She laughed and agreed. We found a rock that formed a sort of table. As I set up, Annie threw pebbles in the shallow water and told me her story.

Annie Jenkins

"You have to be a saint on this Diet. How else could you do it? It is very hard to deny one's self the desires of the heart. My desires were always food, and the more the better. I placed food above everything: my health, my family, even God. Food is what I worshipped. I didn't realize it at the time, but I devoted a huge amount of my life to food. I read food magazines for new recipes, shopped all over town for the best cut of meat, the freshest vegetables, the crustiest bread. I took pains to prepare beautiful meals. I threw elaborate dinner parties. I took pride in the fact that I always made homemade pastries for every bake sale and food drive. I loved to cook, and I loved food, and it showed.

"I was seventy-five pounds overweight when I started the Rice Diet. I am really short, so seventy-five pounds looked like a hundred on me. I looked like a ball, perfectly round. When I look at pictures of me from that time, I am so embarrassed. I looked like something out of a carnival. I had a balloon face with a fringe of bangs and poofy sides which made me look even rounder. My hands and feet looked tiny, and my body looked like one of those inflatable clown dolls that you knock down and they come back up. Of course I am always wearing black in the pictures because I thought it made me look thinner!

"I gave up my old life when I became a Ricer. I stopped reading cooking magazines. I stopped going to grocery stores and farmer's markets. I stopped cooking. It was hard to do that because I really enjoy cooking, but cooking makes food even more pleasurable and, as Dr. Kempner always said, 'food is pleasurable enough' for fat people. We don't have to enhance the experience of it.

"I stayed on rice and fruit until I couldn't stand it anymore. That was about forty days, the same amount of time that Christ spent in the wilderness. After that testing period, I was free from the perils of food cravings. I have never gone back to my old way of life. My family doesn't know what to think. They are angry because I am not the same old chief cook and bottle washer I once was. I no longer worship food or associate with those who do.

"I got to goal weight, and I intend to maintain it. The only way I know of doing that is to follow the Rice Diet. It works. When I follow the Diet I feel good. I feel cool, calm, and collected. I feel that I am living an authentic life. Without the Diet, I would feel lost in the secular world. I am devoted to the Rice Diet."

Annie smiled at me and then looked away. We sat there a few minutes and looked at the water. A man and a couple of boys sauntered by with a big dog. They chatted with us then moved on. Annie and I walked back to our cars.

Rhonda Beru was a Rice House elder. I had talked to her often because we usually sat at the same table. Rhonda was one of the grandmothers of the Diet program and liked to hover and coo over younger participants. I liked her and called her Ronni, as did most of her friends. She was a widow with grown children and grandchildren, but she never spoke about her family.

I knew she was a self-made millionaire, and she read the stock market pages of several newspapers each day. She had a computer and read the very latest quotes. I was surprised that a woman her age was so computer savvy, but Ronni was full of curiosity and believed in learning new things.

I met Ronni for her interview at the Perkins Library on Duke's main campus. She often went there to read books from a variety of disciplines. A high school dropout, she spent most of her free time educating herself. She was forced to quit school when she was sixteen because her father became ill.

I found her in one of the carrels, surrounded by books and magazines. She waved as I approached her and told me how thin I looked. Pleased, I sat down. We talked about things in general for a good twenty minutes. Clearly, Ronni did not like to be rushed, and I wasn't in any hurry. A young man came to the door, but we shooed him away. Ronnie took off her glasses and laid them aside. Rubbing the bridge of her nose, she began her tale.

Rhonda Beru

"I believe in the infallibility of the Rice Diet. Everything that Dr. Kempner said is true. You can free yourself from the effects of bad health and get off all medications by following the Diet. I am seventy-nine years old and am disease free. I take no medications, and my blood pressure, cholesterol, insulin, and weight are all within the normal range. I have no arthritis or pain anywhere. My mental abilities are still functioning up to par, and I just feel good. I wake up in the morning with a sense of power and health. I know it will be a good day because I am capable of handling anything that comes along. I am this way because I adhere to the Diet and have done so for twenty-five years.

"When I started the Rice Diet, I was the typical American housewife. I served meat and potatoes every night for dinner with a wedge of iceberg lettuce slathered with blue cheese dressing. Iceberg lettuce was the only vegetable of the meal. I always served two desserts, usually a fruit pie and a layer cake. Breakfast on the weekends was bacon and eggs, or French toast, or maybe an omelet. Eating like that, I naturally got fat. So did everyone in my family, but we all thought it was normal. Everyone we knew was a little plump.

"We lived in Ohio at the time. One day my husband dropped

dead of a heart attack. He was forty-six. One moment he was here, and the next moment he wasn't. We didn't really think he was that ill. He had heart disease but was on medication and a modified diet. He died anyway. Obviously, the medicine and low-fat diet weren't enough to save him. My oldest son got heart disease too, and I was diagnosed with diabetes. That is how I came to the Rice House. My diabetes was out of control and overtaxing my kidneys.

"At the Rice House I changed my life, and now I devote myself to the Diet. I was converted to the Diet by a good friend of mine. Not only does it save the body, but it saves the soul. I was a nervous wreck before I came to Durham. I thought I was taking care of myself and my family, but I wasn't. I thought I was a good religious person. I believed in God and went to church and volunteered in the community and read the Bible and prayed. Boy, did I pray. 'Please, God, deliver me from my curse of obesity and help me to stick to a diet.' God never heard my prayers. It wasn't until I went to the Rice House that God heard me, and I heard God. I used to say that I believed in God, but He didn't believe in me. Now I know that He does believe in me and He has shown it by granting me thinness and the gift of the Rice Diet.

"I have had no desire for forbidden food since the first time I was in Durham. That burden has been lifted. I just feel blessed every day that I have the opportunity to live and follow the Diet."

Ronni clapped her hands together, stood up, and started to gather her books. I looked at her closely. She did look like the picture of health and moved like a much younger woman. Obviously, the Rice Diet worked for her. She leaned over and repeated the Kempner chant: "Do it, do it, do it." I watched her go back to the stacks, and then I took the stairs back down to the first floor.

Doris Knott was such a kick to interview that I let her keep on talking after I ran out of tape. I liked Doris because she had the enthusiasm of a true believer. I met her at the Center for Living, where she often exercised, but she was a born-again Ricer who lived the Diet and preached its virtues to others. People considered Doris some kind of nut because she would go from church to church in Durham testifying about the healing powers of the Rice

Diet. She was around fifty years old and the owner of a chain of nationally known health spas. Divorced with a grown son, she had residences in Phoenix and Durham.

Doris and I went to church together one Sunday, then walked to the Rice House for a feast of fried chicken, potato pancakes, and salad. The Rice House had the best food on Sunday, and the best meal of the day was lunch. Everyone showed up for that meal. If you were late, you didn't get any fried chicken and had to wait a week for it to reappear. The chicken wasn't actually fried but baked (without skin) at a high enough temperature to brown it. The potato pancakes weren't fried but baked without eggs or flour. Still, they tasted better than anything else served there.

At the dining table, Doris chatted with old friends and made new ones. As the waitress brought in our plates, she bowed her head and said a prayer. All of us, even the waitress, followed Doris's lead. After the meal was over and most of the Ricers had gone, Doris went back to the kitchen to thank the cook for the meal and to acknowledge all of the waitresses. It was a nice touch, and they seemed to appreciate it. I set up my stuff in a little anteroom off the front parlor. Doris came in and sat down in a chair. I asked her to tell me how she felt about the Rice Diet. She smiled, put her hand to her heart, and began.

Doris Knott

"My religion has deep southern, and I guess you would say Baptist, roots. That's why I felt so at home in Durham. My late father was from Canada, but my mother is from Mississippi. I remember going each summer to my grandparents' house for vacation and going to church on Sundays. We never went to church back home, but at my grandparents', it was a requirement. The church was plain and simple, the pews hard and worn, but I loved it there. I found a luxury of spirit in that little church. It was in Pinecrest, Mississippi, in July of 1964, that I found God and took Jesus Christ as my personal savior and was baptized in the holy waters of that church. I was cleansed, and every spot on my soul was removed, and even though I was fat, I knew God loved me in spite of it. God loved me. I felt so good; so purposeful. It wasn't until twenty years later, when I walked into the Rice House, that I felt that way again. I knew that God still loved me. I knew that He knew me personally. He knew my name. And together, we would get me on the right path to salvation, to life. That's how I got to Durham and the Rice House. God brought me.

"I am a worshipper of the Rice Diet and of God. To me there is no difference. God certainly must have inspired Dr. Kempner to create the Rice Diet. The Diet has healed so many people and continues its work. It has cured me of my disease of obesity. I am a walking testimony to the power of the Diet and to the glory of God. You see, if you petition God long and hard enough He will show you the way. For me, that way is the Rice Diet."

I looked up from my notes and saw a waitress standing just outside the room. She had a white paper bag with Doris's name on it. Doris looked up, smiled, and motioned her in. The bag had leftover chicken in it. I could smell it. I thanked Doris for her interview and walked her to her car. She took my hand and thanked me for the opportunity to share the message of the Rice Diet.

Alicia Adams did not share Doris's evangelical roots. She came to the Rice Diet with a New Age background. I met Alicia through a friend of a friend. I had never seen her at the Rice House, nor did I know anything about her, but I met her at the home of a fellow Ricer one evening with a group of other women. According to my friend, the gathering was intended to bring women interested in body image issues together. My guess would be that would include every woman in America, and probably the world.

I hit it off with Alicia because she was from Santa Cruz, and I had spent time there. We liked the same bookstores and shops. She was a thirty-nine-year-old psychotherapist and Reiki master, and the quintessential Californian—tanned, blonde, with beautiful white teeth. She was born in Los Angeles, but grew up in Marin County. Alicia wasn't the name she was born with, but rather the one she gave herself after losing weight. She was a strong believer in the human potential movement and thought that spirituality was central to her life.

One morning, I got a phone call from Alicia asking if I would like to meet her for bagels and coffee. I agreed, and we spent a nice hour or so people-watching. We talked about things in general, and then I came right out and asked her why she was a Diet worshipper. What made her convert? She looked down at her uneaten bagel and folded it back up into its paper wrapping. She played with the rim of her coffee cup, but said nothing. Again I asked her to explain it all to me. She looked away, then back at me, and spoke.

Alicia Adams

"I believe that there is a reason for everything. That is how the cosmos works. And the reason we have to go through so much crap and keep repeating the same old mistakes and patterns is that we are just not evolved enough to see them for what they are or to get out of them. When I came to Durham, I was spiritually evolving. I had been to workshops, and I meditated and journaled, I had balance in all areas of my inner and outer life, but hey, I was very, very fat and pissed off about it. No amount of chanting or loving my spirit within could get me over it. The big *it* was me, my fat. It wasn't until I found the Rice Diet that I stopped struggling with becoming and just became. I experienced illumination. I followed the Diet, lost weight, and felt very clear and pure. Not one stone in my life was unturned. It was as though a huge wind blew through me and got rid of all of the unnecessary debris.

"Once I became a convert to the Rice Diet, I threw out all of my crystals and candles, tarot card deck, I Ching, books, the works. Who needed them? I had the Rice Diet. I was free. I realized that it was not only the food that was blocking me and making me fat, but also my incessant search for something more in my life. I needed more food, more sex, more drugs, more books, more exercise, more spiritual retreats, more time—always more time. I have been to Mecca, and I have walked the path of St. James. I have even been to Lourdes, but I still found myself fat and in spiritual longing. I ate well before the Rice Diet. I was a total vegetarian, but obviously, I ate too much. I thought I was eating moderately and just to the point of fullness, but I wasn't. I exercised aerobically for an hour four days a week, plus walked everywhere, but that wasn't enough either. I was a very healthy person, but I was also a very fat person. It is like Dr. Kempner said: 'We are different people, and what works for others will not work for us.' I had to really, really starve and exercise to the point of exhaustion to lose the weight. That and cut myself off from my undisciplined friends.

"My conversion to the Diet really ticked off all of my old friends because they were used to me being this big, fat, accommodating dumb groupie type who went along with anything, but now I am like this goddess. I am serene. I am it. Oh, I believe in God now. A real one. You can find His spirit at the Rice House in Durham, North Carolina."

I loved Alicia's testimony and the conviction with which she spoke of her Diet faith. You can try through prayer and practice, but nothing catapults you to enlightenment like a big drop in weight. I wondered what Buddha would have thought of Alicia's path. We left the bagel shop together, then parted ways. Last I heard, Alicia had opened up a retreat center somewhere in the mountains. I can picture her perched on a rock, surrounded by seekers looking for direction.

Susan Baird was another Ricer who found the true path through the Rice Diet. I met Susan at Lan Tan's Asian cooking school in Durham. Many Ricers go to Lan's to learn how to cook tasty low-fat dishes. Like everyone there, I was trying to figure out a way to be able to eat food that tasted good without many calories. Some dishes were a success and some failed to inspire us. I was standing next to Susan in class, and our job was to chop vegetables. We began talking, and she told me her story and how central the Rice Diet was to her life. Susan was a forty-year-old journalist from St. Paul, Minnesota, and was married with four children. Later on I interviewed her at her home in Durham over tea and the leftover rice balls we'd made in Lan's class.

Susan Baird

"I started the program when it was at the old Rice House on Mangum Street. It was during a routine morning ritual when I got saved. I was sitting on a sofa waiting for the door to the dining room to open so I could go in and have breakfast. Dr. Newborg was passing around some photos of successful Ricers. I took one that looked exactly like me. It was of a woman of around my age, height, and weight. To me, she looked good. She was well-groomed and dressed nicely and was smiling in the photo. Anyone looking at her would say she was a good-looking woman who was making the most of herself despite the fact that she was fat. Then Dr. Newborg pulled out the 'after' photo of her. She was beautiful—not just pretty, but hauntingly beautiful. She was so skinny she looked like someone out of Biafra. She had these skinny, stick-like legs, a very short spiky haircut, and huge, soulful eyes. She reminded me of the fasting saints icons from the Middle Ages. She looked like she was about to ascend into heaven. When I saw Mary's photo that morning I knew that all things were possible. I could be like she was; I could be thin. From that moment on, I called her St. Mary.

"I was a healthy skeptic. I came to the Rice Diet because I had hit bottom and had nowhere else to go. I wasn't a convert immediately like some people. It took me a good three months to actually get the faith of it. It wasn't until I saw Mary's photo that the Diet took root in me. Coincidentally, the day I saw her photo was the day I found my first bone. That is when I started to believe in the transcendent power of the Diet. I took a nap that afternoon, and upon waking, placed my hand on my chest and felt a bone protruding. I thought for sure I had finally broken something, that I had turned over in my sleep and my stressed bones had finally given way. What I had discovered was my own sternum finally surfacing from its deep bed of fat. I had lost enough weight that my bones could be felt. That is when I got the religion of it all. I was a doubting Thomas who needed some proof, some sign that the Rice Diet was the real thing. I walked around all day feeling my sternum and marveling at it. That night as I was getting undressed I found my own hipbones. A few weeks later I saw my collarbone for the first time. I found out from others at the Rice House who had lost a lot of weight that all of them had found their own bones too. Seeing my bone structure emerge was the pivotal moment for me. That beast inside me that demanded more food left. Now I feel peaceful, calm, and satisfied with one bowl of rice and two pieces of fruit. My soul is at rest."

After Susan finished her speech, we looked down at the one remaining rice ball. Without saying a word, she took a knife and carefully divided it in two. She offered one half to me and I took it. I knew that this was most likely all she would eat for dinner and could be all the food she'd have for the day. I felt a little ashamed to take the last of the rice balls. I waited until she ate her half; then I popped mine into my mouth. It tasted divine.

Carol Witherspoon was a seventy-two-year-old Diet worshipper from Rancho Mirage, California, who had spent a lifetime searching for the perfect diet. I met her at the Rice House and spent the day with her as she walked the wall at Duke's east campus, attended step aerobics class, then a Pilates class, and finally a water aerobics class. I couldn't keep up with her and quit exercising after the Pilates torture. Later that evening, we met for a drink at a restaurant near the Rice House. Carol drank mineral water and smoked menthol cigarettes.

I sat and placed my tape recorder on the bar. Nobody even looked around to see what I was doing. By now, all of Durham and most of Chapel Hill was used to seeing me whip out my tape recorder and drop a cassette or two on the bars and floors of public spots. The bartender emptied the dirty ashtray and slid a clean one under Carol's droopy cigarette. In a deep voice she began.

Carol Witherspoon

"The Rice Diet saved my body and my soul. Now I am strong in body and mind and will have to be killed to die. Remember what Dr. Rosati tells us: 'The only way a Ricer can die is in an accident.' We are too strong to go any other way. Fate will have to take us out.

"I met up with some wonderful souls the first day on the Diet. I sat down at a table, and this woman there told me a tale of her journey on the Rice Diet. I watched her as she spoke. Her face was radiant and she had such faith in the Diet that I too wanted to be a true believer. I wanted to be thin in body and full in spirit. I knew the Rice House was the place for me.

"I didn't get salvation right off. Like everything else it takes time, but the wonderful thing about being in Durham on a diet program is, all you have is time. I followed the Diet hour by hour. That was how food obsessed I was. I could only go an hour without desiring it. Then I could go a whole morning without craving something. Finally, after a month on program, I could go a whole twenty-four hours without cheating. That was a miracle to me. I had never been able to stay on a diet or deny myself anything before. I blamed myself for being weak, for lacking willpower. What I really lacked was a religion, the religion of the Rice Diet. Now I can go days without eating, and I don't feel a thing. I don't get hungry, I don't get tired, and I don't get weak. The Rice Diet is it for me. The ultimate. I will follow it until I am killed in a wreck."

After Carol finished she started to cough. The bartender thoughtfully brought over another bottle of mineral water. I thanked him as Carol continued to choke. Finally, she managed to take a sip and looked up to me. Her watery eyes shone like a true believer's. I looked around to see if anyone was listening and several people nodded and raised a glass to Carol. I didn't know if they were Ricers, or dieters, or just thought her talk was entertaining. When I left, Carol was still at the bar.

There are those among us who do not find religion through dieting. Their souls are not saved at the Rice House; instead, they are lost. Ellen Livingston is one of those lost souls of Durham.

I wanted to interview Ellen because she had had a different experience with the Rice Diet than the successful true believers. I knew that there had to be people who didn't succeed at dieting. Many people considered Ellen a failure of the Diet program and used her as a warning to new participants of the dangers and pitfalls that can occur when a Ricer is not vigilant. It frightened me to interview her because I was afraid that I was just like her. I was used to dieting and was becoming immune to the power of Durham.

I interviewed Ellen at the Rice House. Even though she was not on program anymore, she showed up at the Rice House from time to time to see old friends and to participate in social events. She always came in the evening, when the staff was not around.

The dinner crowd had left for the evening. Most of them were heading out to the nearby movie complex. Ellen and I were sitting in the living room. Ricers came by to say hello and invite us to go with them. We politely declined. When the room was empty, I asked Ellen what had happened to her on the Rice Diet. She looked down at her wide lap and folded and unfolded her hands. Finally, she took a deep breath and told me.

Ellen Livingston

"I absolutely believe in the power of the Rice Diet. I believe that it is really a spiritual diet rather than a physical one. It cures the soul as well as the body. I was converted the first month I was in Durham. I started the Rice Diet just like everyone else, with the belief that I would lose my fat, get cured, go home and eat whatever I wanted, and never be fat again. I thought that Dr. Kempner had this supernatural power to wave his hand and cure me.

"You know the formula to cure obesity, don't you? First you must get to goal weight. Then you have to maintain that weight for at least two years. That way, your fat cells will collapse and you won't be fat again. The fat cells never dissolve, but they can collapse. I wanted to be one of the few, one of the chosen that rose above the muck of the fallen world and rang that bell of goal weight. I wanted to be cured. I was like a crusader in the Middle Ages. I focused on weight loss and nothing else. I ate rice and fruit until I thought I was going to die. I would literally choke on it because I was so tired of eating it, but I would do it. I would limit myself to one glass of water a day because I didn't even want water to show up on the scale.

"My family was thrilled. I was losing weight so fast that they actually saw a difference when they came to visit. They were not thrilled that I wouldn't go out to eat with them. They said, 'Come with us. You can have a salad while we eat pizza.' People are absolutely clueless. They have no idea of the power of food, especially to a dieter.

"I was a fanatic on the Diet. I walked to Duke Chapel and back every single morning. Rain, shine, snow, heat, it didn't matter. I felt compelled to be the best dieter. I was full of pride in myself. I guess I started to believe in my own personal willpower rather than the strength of the Rice Diet. I thought I knew more than Dr. Kempner.

"I started to exercise with people from other programs, and they would tell me to lighten up. Tell me destructive stuff like I should be counting fat grams instead of eating rice and fruit. The fallen world is always there to lead you off the path. Even though I told myself that I wasn't listening, I started to take their messages to heart.

"I decided that I could do it myself; I could follow the Diet without going to the Rice House and without paying those doctors' fees. After all, I was a Ricer now, and I knew as much as any of those doctors. How hard could it be to eat rice and fruit on my own? I rented an apartment that had no kitchen, just a hot plate and one of those dorm refrigerators. I got up each morning and walked to the Ninth Street Bakery and had a bowl of oatmeal and an apple.

"At first I felt very smug and virtuous doing it on my own. I would meet other Ricers at the Bakery and have coffee, and I would think of them as foolish for spending all of that cash at the Rice House. Little by little I just got acclimated to the world again. I exercised at the Center For Living, and soon I was eating in their cafeteria. Everything there is low-fat, low-calorie, and low-sodium, but not nearly as low as at the Rice House. Every now and then I would have dinner with friends at Duke Diet and Fitness Center or Structure House. To all the world, I was still a serious dieter, but I wasn't losing any weight. I even started to gain a few pounds.

"Now, forty pounds up and no place to go, I can't go back to the Rice House because I would feel like an idiot. I practically told them when I left that they were full of crap, and I could do it on my own. I can't go back to California because I am still too fat. So what do I do? Hang around Durham and wait for another miracle to happen."

Ellen threw up her hands in disgust and pushed back her chair. Other Ricers who had been listening to her story looked away. Nobody wanted to acknowledge that some dieters just don't make it, don't get to goal weight. Ellen's story reminded them that some people do fail and thinness isn't a guarantee.

Her story scared me too. I didn't want to end up like her and keep my life in a perpetual holding pattern in Durham. I wanted to have a commando raid on my obesity. Hit the ground running, get into the Rice House, lose the weight, and get out as fast as possible. Ellen read my expression and looked me straight in the eye. I was the first one to blink and look down at the table. She leaned over, patted my hand, and whispered in my ear that she was sure I would reach goal, that I was one of the lucky ones. I mumbled my thanks and looked up to watch Ellen leave with another Ricer.

I met Julie Williams at an Overeaters Anonymous meeting in Chapel Hill. Many Ricers go to that particular meeting because it is filled with people from different diet programs and there is a kind of "comparison of diets" chat after the meeting. Julie was a young woman from Los Angeles, California. She was taking a year off between college and graduate school. Her plan was to get a master's degree in Business Administration from Duke University.

Like most of the Ricers I've interviewed, Julie was very self-aware and saw herself clearly. I met her at a bar in Chapel Hill for a preliminary interview. We talked and exchanged phone numbers and promised to keep in touch to shore up each other's resolve to lose weight. I saw her from time to time around Durham and Chapel Hill, but we never talked much. I think she was embarrassed that she'd shared so much that night or was ashamed that she hadn't lost any weight since our first meeting.

One day I got a call from Julie requesting an interview. I met her at the student union at Duke. She walked from her apartment to Duke Chapel several times a week, and the student union was her halfway point. We arrived at the same time, got our drinks, and found an available table. The noise level was high, and I wasn't sure if I would be able to record clearly. I took out my notebook and pen and Julie began.

Julie Williams

"I guess you could call me a sinner any way you look at it. I started the Rice Diet with such good intentions. I have been on Duke Diet and Fitness Center and Structure House and my family and myself were really at a loss as to where I should go next. I lose the same eighty pounds over and over again. Sometimes I can keep the weight off for two or three years, but usually, I gain it back within five to six months.

"The Rice Diet was different than any diet I had ever been on, and I loved it immediately. I felt good and almost holy on the Diet. Eating rice and fruit functions as a purification rite, and after going through six weeks of that, I did feel cleansed. I had no desire for any kind of food other than Rice House food. I felt great and I wasn't hungry. I was converted. The Rice Diet was it for me. I loved it. The simplicity of it appealed to something deep within me. I felt like a monk, or a pilgrim, or one of those beggars in India who walk around the country with their alms bowls. I was satisfied. I had reached nirvana. I had no desires, no lusts, no longing. I had no sex while on the Diet either. I thought that sex would pollute my body. I was born again as a virgin. It was as though my promiscuous past had been erased. I felt like a new person in a new body.

"I ate every meal in the Rice House. I ate at the same time every day. I exercised every day too. I wrote in my journal. I attended all Rice House meetings. I turned in my urine samples. I hung around an older group of women who were faithful to the Rice Diet. We went shopping together, and they just fawned over me. I felt so much love from them. They told me how awful their lives had been before the Rice Diet, how ill they had been before they lost weight. They were miracle tales, I guess. I just loved hearing them.

"I almost got to goal weight, but then something happened. My mother got ill, and I had to go back home. The Rice House staff told me that it would be a mistake to go home, but I felt all of this pressure. I am an only child and my parents are divorced, so who was going to take care of my mother? My mother had colon cancer, and I had to be there for the surgery and recovery and all of the treatments.

"I went home with the best of intentions. I bought a rice steamer and lugged it around everywhere. Ate oatmeal for breakfast and rice and fruit for lunch and dinner. I would not drive because I needed to walk. The weight just came back, and it came back fast. I was taking care of my mother, scheduling her medications and doctors' appointments, trying to figure out the medical insurance and hospital bills, dealing with my father and my grandmother, and trying to get into graduate school. It was a horrible time in my life, but I still had the sanity that the Rice Diet provides. Then one day my faith just deserted me, and I was alone in a house full of forbidden food. I realized that I was no better than anybody else, I wasn't any purer, or stronger, or better. I might as well eat as the rest of the world eats, because I was a part of the world. From that moment, the weight rushed back on.

"I am back in Durham again. I want to lose around sixty-five pounds before school, but I don't know if I can go back to the Rice House. I have this deep longing for it, but I feel like I have failed everyone there. I feel like a sinner."

Julie pulled out a cigarette and leaned over and allowed the bartender to light it for her. I guess since she was no longer on the Rice Diet and losing weight, she believed that her body was no longer a temple and no longer pure. Now she was free to indulge in all her old vices. I stayed a couple of hours and drank seltzer water as I watched her knock back tequila shooters. Convinced that she was not fit to be behind the wheel, I drove Julie to her apartment and waited until she was safely in the door.

For the Diet to be truly effective for many Ricers, it must become like a religion. Followers must perform their religious duties: adhering to the food restrictions of the Diet and exercising on a daily basis. The requirements of dieting become rituals and are performed with solemn devotion. Those who do really well on the Diet become worshippers. They are considered examples of people who live right and are rewarded with weight loss and weight maintenance. Those souls who lose the intensity of the Diet are viewed by the greater dieting community as sinners, warnings of what can happen if you are not mindful of the Diet.

I was not converted to the Rice Diet as deeply as those I have interviewed, but I do praise it. I guess my faith in the Diet is like my faith in everything else, a continuum between doubt and belief. That belief was strong enough to make me sell everything, drive across the country, and follow the advice of an old man who spoke only in parables. It was strong enough to make me eat nothing but rice and fruit and lose a hundred pounds. Yet I never felt saved in the sense that I felt peaceful and content. It is not my nature to feel so. I remain restless and easily bored, and my cycle of weight gains and weight losses reflects my character flaws. I see the Diet as a job that must be performed without any hope of retirement. I view it as an occupation, not a religion.

ten

The Occupation of Dieting

Those of us who are lifer Ricers, who have been on the Rice Diet for years, view ourselves as professionals and leaders in diet culture. Many of us consider dieting an occupation rather than a religion, especially after the initial motivation to lose weight has worn off. We workers of the Rice Diet are not new to Durham, nor are we the true believers in the Rice Diet or enthusiasts like the beginning dieters. The good news of the novices is old news to us.

Male Dieters especially view the Rice Diet as a profession. They are recognized by Dieters and doctors alike as superior weight losers. They have mastered the skills of the dieting profession. They possess the same characteristics as do professionals in any other field: they have expertise, autonomy, commitment, and identification with other dieters, and they uphold the standards and ethics of dieting. They see themselves in Durham as at the top of their profession, where all their years of dieting attempts, successful weight losses, and rebounding weight gains have led them.

Those of us who work the program have the expertise. We have been on many diets. We are separated from novice dieters because we can come and go as we please at the Rice House. Sometimes we do not even have our meals at the Rice House, but get them delivered.

Technique reflects the working knowledge of an occupation and is passed on from one worker to another through experience and habit. We work the Diet and learn the two techniques vital to doing so: the ability to get along with others, and the skills to regulate food intake and the body's response to that food.

To be good Ricers, we must get along with the Rice House staff, the doctors, and fellow Ricers. The Rice Diet is the only diet program in Durham that does not have a formal introduction or sanctioned initiation period. All of Durham's other programs—the Center for Living, the Duke Diet and Fitness Center, Structure House—have introductory classes, information packets full of helpful hints, instructions, maps of Durham, lists of social activities, and meetings of new participants. These programs initiate each dieter and provide guidelines for appropriate behavior. The Rice Diet staff, on the other hand, instructs us to show up at the Rice House in the morning. That is all the information we receive. Each of us must make our way through Ricer culture on our own. Since there is no official instruction for new Ricers, we have developed oral traditions which address informal initiations.

The most important step in the occupation of dieting is the selection of a co-worker. This is vital to mastering the technique of getting along with others. If you select a co-worker who consistently cheats on the Diet and disregards directives from the staff, you fail at the occupation of dieting. When we begin the Rice Diet, the old association with food breaks. Something or someone must take over the role that food has played. The staff encourages the buddy system, but does not arrange partnerships. Dr. Kempner felt that people, when left to their own devices, would find what they needed.

For the Rice Diet staff and participants, the world is black or white, right or wrong. There is no in-between; one is either a serious dieter or one is not. To discover the character of a new dieter, old Ricers administer a series of pranks. All Ricers, including staff, like to believe that everyone at the Rice House is of equal standing, yet they are not. The Rice House—especially the staff—thinks of itself in terms of a family. In reality, like any other work environment, it is an arena of changing tensions and resolutions. Pranks reveal these elements and are crucial to the developing techniques of getting along with others. These pranks, or practical jokes, play the same roles that they would in any other job. A newcomer must learn to fit in with the older, more experienced group. It is an ongoing process.

Pranks between unequals are the most common ones found in diet culture. They are a way to teach new dieters their place in the greater dieting community. Joel Fishbine, a forty-three-year-old businessman, was pranked during his first tour of the Rice House. I interviewed Joel on Valentine's Day at a coffee shop in Chapel Hill. Joel wanted to be away from the Rice House for the interview; he didn't want other Ricers to overhear his tale, even though many of them had already told me about the prank played on him. I suppose he was embarrassed by it.

When I got to the coffee shop, Joel was already seated, reading his newspaper. He looked up at me over his reading glasses and motioned me to his table. The waitress brought me a cup of coffee, which I drank immediately. Joel continued reading his paper. On my third coffee refill, after he had finished the daily crossword puzzle, Joel put away the paper, folded his hands, and asked me what exactly I wanted of him. Did I have any specific questions in mind? I told him that I wanted to know about pranks played on Ricers. I had heard a lot of stories at the Rice House but wanted his version.

Joel smiled, rubbed his forehead, and began to recall.

Joel Fishbine

"When I was a new recruit about a decade ago, I used to get a lot of practical jokes played on me by the old guys. There used to be a table of guidos who used to really give it to me; they just wouldn't let up. Well, I learned something from those old farts. I learned the official rules of the Diet from the staff, but understood the real rules of the program from those guys.

"I lived off rice and fruit for six weeks and I was tired, starved, and a little testy. I had lost all of my social graces. In fact, I was just plain rude and didn't give a damn about respecting other people. I didn't think I needed co-workers or buddies because I wasn't in

Durham to make friends; I was there to lose weight. And who were those old farts to tell me how to behave? At this low point in my life, these old Ricers started to lay traps for me. I guess they were trying to see what I was made of, or even if I could take a joke. I was a bit temperamental.

"They pranked me on a food request. This was the old days at the Rice House on Mangum, where we used to get chicken. It was my day to get chicken. I had been to Dr. Newborg and must have argued my case pretty good, because she gave me the permission slip. I took it into the kitchen and gave it to them and could hardly wait to taste meat for the first time in weeks. It was a Sunday morning too, so that meant chicken, a potato pancake, and salad for lunch. It would be a feast.

"I went for a long jog, got a newspaper, and walked back to the Rice House. I sat down at my usual table and filled out the request slip for my lunch. And guess what? The food never showed up. I went up to the door of the kitchen and asked the manager, 'What gives? Where's my chicken?' He told me that they had run out of chicken and I could have rice and fruit or nothing at all, and to make my decision fast because the dining room was getting crowded. I was so mad I thought I was going to punch him in the face. Instead, I just got a box of shredded wheat and a couple of oranges and left. As I walked by that one table everyone just burst out laughing and looked right at me. I knew they had screwed with me and were in cahoots with the staff. I was so pissed at first, but then I realized that they were just telling me to lighten up and quit being such an asshole. I was taking my fat self too seriously. I guess you could call it my initiation."

Satisfied with his story, Joel waved the waitress over and paid the bill. He looked pleased with himself and even proud that he'd been pranked. To him, it was a badge of honor, a mark of acceptance into the community. I laughed out loud at his story and asked him if he was still in touch with those pranksters. "Yes," he said, "they are my close friends."

Joel stood up when I left and told me he would see me at the Rice House. When I got to the door, I turned back and saw him scribbling on his newspaper. He was probably working the jumble puzzle. I figured this was how he spent his days on the Rice Diet—hanging around coffee shops drinking cup after cup of decaf.

Debra Seldors got a message from her Diet co-workers also. I met Debra at a Ricer celebration party for the Super Bowl. I hadn't really had a conversation with her before. I knew she was from Chicago, was a litigation attorney for an international law firm, and was single but living with someone she'd met while on program. I was intimidated by Debra. She was young, successful, confident, and very determined to get to goal weight and get out of Durham. She didn't seem to have any doubts about her ability to reach goal or to maintain it.

After an introductory meeting at the party, we went off to another room for the interview. She didn't have much time, and I assured her that the interview wouldn't take long. Twice during the interview her beeper went off, but Debra kept on reciting her story as if she wasn't aware of the interruption.

Debra Seldors

"I am an old hand at the Rice House now. I have been here off and on for eight visits, and when I show up it is old home week. Now it is all routine for me, and I get right back into the work of the Rice Diet. I go to the rice and fruit table for a purge that lasts at least three weeks. I try to stay on rice and fruit the whole time, but just can't seem to do it as well as the first time I was here. The Rice Diet is just like any other job: you learn it, you work it, and then when you get off work, you go and do something else. I consider being back home as being off work from the Rice Diet.

"The first time I was here I thought of myself as different from the rest of the crew. I thought I knew everything: I was educated, wealthy, ambitious, and cultured. In short, I was a snob. I looked down my nose at those Dieters who I thought just weren't up to snuff—those older ones who just come and go as they please at the Rice House and don't get in any kind of trouble if they don't show up for meals. I mean, what is the point? Why do they hang around if they aren't willing to diet? I would have nothing to do with them.

"Then one day around noon, one of the ladies from that group came over to my table for a chat. I was suspicious at first, but then opened up. I was miserable because I just couldn't gag down the rice anymore. It had no taste. She nodded and told me that she had something that would put a little flavor in the rice without sodium or calories. She told me that it was perfectly legal and that Dr. Newborg endorsed the product. Then she pulled a bottle of Tennessee Sunshine Hot Pepper Sauce out of her handbag and gave it to me. She put it right in front of me on the table. I grabbed it and shook it all over my boiled rice. She told me to keep the bottle and excused herself from the table. At dinner, I used the sauce again and could actually swallow the rice. The next day at weigh-in, I had put on five pounds! It was the Sunshine. When I went in to the dining room for breakfast somebody had taped up a sign that read 'Tennessee Sunshine is Verboten.' Those women had screwed with me, set me up. Tennessee Sunshine is loaded with sodium. I was pranked and everyone knew it. The whole Rice House was laughing at me. For weeks people called me Sunshine every time I walked into the dining room. To this day, I still get bottles of Sunshine sent to me for Christmas."

Debra got up, thanked me for the interview, and went off to join some of her friends for a run through Duke Forest before I had time to formulate a response. She was out the door the moment I clicked off the tape recorder. As I was packing my gear, another Ricer, Leslie Bennett, stuck her head into the room and asked if I would interview her sometime. Apparently she and some other Ricers had overhead Debra's story. Leslie had a story of her own to tell. We agreed to meet at a later time, somewhere outside the Rice House.

I looked forward to interviewing Leslie. I knew her very well and sitting down with her would be as comfortable as talking to an old friend. Leslie was the owner of a chain of nationally known weight-loss centers. Everyone on the Rice Diet—including me—had probably been a client of those centers at one time or another. I was surprised that Leslie hadn't gone to one of her own centers to lose weight, but she told me that because she had such a large amount of weight to lose, she came to the Rice Diet instead. The Rice Diet is the only one that works for her. She believes that everyone has a different dieting style and no single diet will work for all people.

I interviewed Leslie outside a bagel shop in Durham. We sat at one of the few tables scattered around and watched Duke students ride by on their bicycles. She sipped mineral water while I drank coffee with cream and sugar. We split a dry bagel. Leslie didn't consider the bagel to be cheating on the Diet because she didn't eat the whole thing. She said she was only eating it as part of a social ritual of food and conversation.

Leslie Bennett

"The Rice Diet is my place of business, and my job is losing weight. Dr. Kempner told me that years ago, and he was right. Maintaining my weight is a full-time job and I do it by returning to the Rice House periodically and becoming more proficient at dieting. It doesn't get easier, but it gets to be a habit and that makes it better. Coming back to the Rice House keeps me in touch with my profession and stops weight gain. Also, it is the only place where I can totally focus on my job, which is to lose weight, without interruptions. I have made a lot of friends here, and I enjoy the whole experience. My friends help facilitate my weight loss. They encourage me and usually set a good example. It wasn't always that way.

"The first couple of times I was on program, I was in attack mode. I would fly in to Durham, go to the Rice House, sit by myself at the rice and fruit table, gobble down my little piles of food, and then run out the door for a seven-mile hike through Duke Forest. I didn't have time for anything else. I wouldn't talk to other Ricers at meals, I wouldn't go with them to the movies or on any other outings, and I wouldn't hang around on the front porch and chat. I just wanted to lose weight, get in shape, and get the hell out of Durham. I also wanted to be left alone. I thought I could be cured of my obesity, and once thin, never look back. Now I know that isn't possible, but then I was young and arrogant.

"The ladies of the Rice House had invited me on several outings:

shopping, cooking classes at Lan's, the movies, plays at Duke, the American Dance Festival, even a trip to the beach, but I wouldn't have any of it. It wasn't that I didn't like them; I didn't even want to take the effort and time to get to know them. I didn't want to get involved. Time after time I would politely but firmly turn down all invitations. I was relieved when they stopped asking.

"One day I showed up for weigh-in and literally leaped on the scale. I was sure I was going to get to the forty-pound midway point of my weight loss plan. I was losing weight like a champion dieter and was secretly gloating every time I got on the scale and had a three- to-four-pound drop. The ladies that hung out together only lost three to four pounds a week. I felt superior to them. The staff treated me like some golden child because I was such a good little dieter. They loved to tell the new people just coming on program how much weight I had lost in such a short amount of time. That morning, I got on the scale and instead of losing weight, I had gained four pounds. Right then Dr. Kempner came by and pointed his bony finger at me and asked, 'Did you lose?' No, I hadn't lost; in fact, I had gained. There was no explanation for the weight gain. It wasn't my period and I hadn't cheated. Then I looked over, and those gals were all smirking at me. Everywhere I looked people were smirking, even the staff. Then I knew they had messed with the calibration of the scales. It was their way of saying 'up yours.' That's when I got some humility and began to blend in more, be more of a team player."

Leslie smiled and picked up the last of her bagel. She wasn't proud of being on the receiving end of a prank as Joel Fishbine had been. Instead, she seemed sort of amazed by it—not by the prank itself, but rather by her initial insensitivity to other Ricers.

After we have been on the Diet for a while the pranks lessen, but occasionally there will be a prank played between equals. It is a way to remind us of who we are and what we are supposed to be doing in Durham. Karen Reeves was a target of one of these pranks. I met Karen at a Durham Bulls baseball game. I had seen her around the Rice House and a couple of times at the Center for Living, but I didn't associate with her or her friends because they were much younger than I was. Karen was very pretty and looked about average in weight to me. I knew she had been very large when she started the Diet, but I hadn't seen her then. Several of us decided to go to the Bulls game, and I ended up sitting next to Karen. She agreed to an interview and I met her later at her apartment.

I was surprised when Karen's boyfriend answered the door. I'd assumed that she lived alone. I also assumed that her boyfriend was another man I had seen her with, not this one. After introductions were made, her boyfriend excused himself, and Karen and I were alone in the living room. She brought out the usual Ricer offerings of shredded wheat squares, rice cakes, orange slices, and herbal tea. As she poured the tea she began talking.

Karen Reeves

"The first time I was on program, I did so well. I was new to Durham and the Rice Diet, and I was such a believer in the entire program, especially in Dr. Kempner and Dr. Newborg. I thought of Kempner as this god of diet culture and Newborg as his gentler, female persona. You could approach Newborg, not Kempner. I was the teacher's pet of the Rice Diet staff. I would be the first one in the Rice House each morning for weigh-in. I got there even before most of the staff showed up. I was the first person on the scale, the first one to turn in a urine bottle, the first one in the dining room, and the first one out for a walk. I even wore my name tag every single day. I lost weight like you wouldn't believe, and so fast—forty-five pounds in the first couple of months on program—and I looked good too. When I first went to the Rice House I was a gorilla. I was this huge lumpy thing with a mop of over-permed and processed hair: a mess. I worked very hard to lose weight and to look good and after a few months, I was looking fabulous.

"I made a lot of friends at the Rice House, and we did everything together: went to movies, shopping, had makeovers, took cooking classes, exercise classes, and had more fun than I ever had in my life. I loved it. When I made my hundred-pound weight loss, the whole Rice House was happy. All of my friends were so proud when they put my name up there on the Century Board. That's the board where they put your name once you drop a hundred pounds. Everyone who walks in the Rice House can read it and see who has dropped a ton of weight. Everyone congratulated me. I was like a symbol of the potency of the Diet. I was a winner.

"It is strange, but from that moment on, I just started to lose the intensity to adhere to the Diet. I no longer had this burning desire to be thin. Also, I had proved to myself and the rest of the Rice House that I could lose weight. I guess I just thought I could go the rest of the way to goal without the help of the Rice Diet. I wanted to look good and be normal, and to me, after a hundred-pound loss, I was normal. To the rest of the world, and especially to the Rice House doctors, I was still morbidly obese, but I could now buy clothes in any store, not just specialty shops. I felt thin and I just started to drift. I would cheat a little here and there, then not show up for morning weigh-in. I would forget to turn in a urine sample, that sort of thing. My friends would try to talk to me and get me pumped up again, even Dr. Newborg tried to counsel me. Nothing worked. My weight loss stopped, and I even put on a pound or two. Then one day I walked into the Rice House and saw that my name on the Century Board had been taken off and repositioned upside down. I knew then that I was losing my status and if I didn't shape up, I would be kicked out of the Rice House for good. It was like getting a warning from your boss because you show up to work late for too many mornings. I knew that I had to get a hold of myself."

I couldn't imagine Karen ever straying from the Diet. To me she was the epitome of the perfect dieter. I guess after we have been dieting for a long time, all of us begin to drift.

Sharon Ward got a prank played on her by her closest friends at the Rice House, though they never admitted it. I had known Sharon for a long time and thought a lot of her. Lots of people thought she was too New Age because she would often tell them that their aura was all wrong, or inform them that they were living out some agenda from a previous life. I thought Sharon was sweet and funny and pleasant to be around. We went many places together.

Sharon owned a cruise line and had residences on both coasts. She was divorced and had a grown daughter who was the acting chief executive officer of her company. I interviewed Sharon at her wonderfully and artfully decorated apartment right across from the Rice House. It was filled with icons and affirmations painted directly on the white walls. Sharon took out her magic marker and wrote a note to herself on the wall whenever she got inspired. I'm sure that her landlord didn't appreciate Sharon's self-expression, but I found it amusing.

I balanced myself on one of Sharon's ornately designed floor pillows and put my tape recorder and notebook on the polished wood floor. Sharon sat across from me, legs folded beneath her. She closed her eyes and bowed her head. For a moment, I thought she was going to pray or break into a chant. My knees ached and I wanted to uncross my legs. Sharon said nothing and kept her head down. Finally, I couldn't take it anymore. I unbent my legs, rolled over, slid the giant pillow under my back, and propped myself up in a sitting position. Sharon looked up, stretched her arms high over her head, inhaled deeply, and held her breath. When her arms began their descend, she slowly exhaled.

Sharon Ward

"I am a born dieter. I have been doing it all of my life. My mother was fat, my grandmother was fat, and both of my sisters are fat. All of the men in my family are beanpoles. It is the women who carry the weight. I was born to diet, just like people were born into trades back in history. My trade is dieting.

"I have been a Ricer for fourteen years. I know what it is about, I know how to work it, I know what pitfalls there are, and what type of people to avoid. I also know when it is time to return to the Rice House—when I try to get up and my butt sticks to the chair.

"When I show up in Durham I sit at the same table with the same people and eat the same food. It is the familiarity and the monotony of the place that makes it so successful. There is an unwritten code of behavior that applies to all of us at the Rice House, whether we know it or not. We learn the rules or we don't make it through the program. The currency of the Rice House is food. To us, food, especially when we are dieting, is the most important thing in life. Sharing food with other Ricers is considered good social behavior at the table. This sharing is forbidden by the staff, because each of us is in a different stage of the Diet. Some of us are still on rice and fruit, some are on vegetables, some get more food and some get less. The food at the Rice House is never measured out, but sort of portioned. Somebody's share may look a little bigger or better than another person's. Somebody's fruit may be riper. Somebody's salad may be fresher, that sort of thing. I had to learn of all of this the hard way.

"My first time on program went really well. I met some nice friends. We always ate together and walked together after meals. We would pool our food resources and divvy them up among us according to the degree of hunger at the table. We didn't consider this cheating per se, because we were still eating the proper food of the Rice Diet and we were eating it in the Rice House, we were just sharing a little food with friends. Sometimes I was hungrier than someone else, and a chicken bone with a little meat on it would appear on my plate. I was on vegetables at the time, so I wasn't allowed meat and I really appreciated that little bit of chicken flesh. I, in turn, would order the extra freebies that you get at the Rice House—raw onions, salad dressing, tomato sauce—and share them with my table mates. Not everybody knows about the freebies, but if you ask for them, the waitress will usually bring some to you. For some reason, I started to get greedy. My appetite picked up and I was hungry all of the time. I reached over a couple of times and pulled some chicken off a friend's plate. I did it without asking. I didn't really care what they thought. They'd shared with me before, so what difference did it make if I took some of their food without asking?

"The day Dr. Newborg let me have chicken was a big day for me. Everyone was happy for me. Then they brought my chicken and it was the wet kind with tomatoes and onions. That sloppy kind that I didn't want. What I wanted was the crispy kind that tasted like fried chicken. I was really disappointed and voiced it pretty loudly. Nobody said a word and then one of the waitresses came out from the kitchen and said I had a phone call. I got up from the table and went into the other room for the phone, and when I got back they had taken my chicken away. Even my placemat was gone! I learned never to complain again."

There are some Ricers who actually play pranks on the Rice House staff and get away with it. Dennis Kota was one of those characters. For the most part, his pranks were merely annoying rather than hurtful. Dennis saw himself as a good prankster, and he enjoyed the reaction he got when one of his pranks was successfully executed.

I was a bit wary of Dennis because I didn't know if he was kidding me when he said he wanted me to interview him or setting me up for one of his jokes. I met him at the Rice House for the interview and waited for him in the parlor. He was talking to some of his buddies and making the rounds. He walked over, plopped down next to me on the faded sofa, folded his massive arms behind his head, and, with a twinkle in his eye, began.

Dennis Kota

"I have been around the Rice House for years. I first came here when I was eighteen and right out of high school. I know just about everything there is to know about the Diet. I can work it well, and I can work it fast. I associate with the superior dieters: those guys who can really drop the weight. I stay away from the women because most of them aren't really here to diet, they are just running away from home and all of their problems. They never want to leave Durham, so they don't lose as much weight. Me, I want to lose weight as fast as I can and leave.

"The most important thing about the Rice House is that there are all of these tensions. I guess it is because we are all fat and pissed off and stuck in Durham eating rice and fruit. All of that is enough to make you want to put your fist through a wall. Plus, there are people from all over the world, with different backgrounds and different socioeconomic situations, so the whole place is ripe for misunderstanding and culture clashes, or learning from others. I guess it all depends on your point of view.

"I started out at the old Rice House on Mangum. It was owned by Tommy Thomas and his family. The Rice House was run differently back then. You had white southern owners, black waitresses, German staff, and a roomful of Jewish dieters. It was an experience. I couldn't understand the waitresses because of their accents, and I couldn't understand Dr. Kempner because of his.

"When I started the Rice Diet I tried to make friends with everyone there, because I knew how important it was to hang with the true dieters and not the slackers who just come to Durham to get laid and party. I wanted to lose weight and get out, so I tried to associate myself with those really successful losers like Danny Thier and Bob Martin. They were the gods of weight loss when I started the program, each one a two-hundred-plus drop from their initial weight. I wanted to be like them. They were always together talking and there was a beautiful girl named Michelle who was often around. She had lost over 170 pounds and was just lovely and so sweet. She was like the pet of the Rice House. I used to sit at their table and I would try to strike up a conversation, but they wouldn't have anything to do with me. It wasn't until I peeled a layer that they would give me the time of day. After I lost around seventy-five pounds, Bob asked me to play golf with them, and that's how we all became friends.

"We used to assess the potential of the incoming dieters and even would bet on who we thought would make it or not. We would rate the women too: this nickel [a woman who weighs 500 pounds] isn't worth it, look at the gorilla, nice little jumboette on the port side, that one needs a buff and shine, that one will never make it. It wasn't not very nice, but we did it anyway. It was a way to pass the time. There was this one guy none of us could stand. His name was Sean, he was from California, and he thought he was God's gift to the world. He had this fake streaked blond hair and tanning bed look about him. Wore these little nylon running shorts all the time. The women loved him, and the doctors thought he was great because he had lost fifty-five pounds in two months; that was the record at the time. We all hated him, but more than that we were pissed at the doctors because they kept singing his praises. Weren't we fast losers also? Didn't we deserve the staff's respect? No, they just ignored us.

"One day we had had enough. I slipped into the portable file boxes, where they have all the medical records and statistics of each patient on the program, and stole Sean's file. And guess what? His name wasn't even Sean. It was Wayne. He wasn't from California, but Pittsburgh, Pennsylvania. His whole story was a line. I stole the file and hid it where nobody would find it for weeks. I didn't destroy it, but I did misplace it. The doctors suspected something, but nobody said a word. Sean/Wayne quit before he got to goal weight."

Some Ricers have played the ultimate prank on Dr. Kempner himself. Perry Swain, an elderly businessman from Dallas, told me the classic prank tale known to all as the Betty Caper. Perry was a constant at the Rice House. Every morning when I went to weigh-in, Perry was sitting on the couch closest to the main door reading a newspaper. He always greeted me with, "Hey, girlie." Perry reminded me of my grandfather. He was always dressed in a starched white shirt and a dark tie. He smelled of Old Spice cologne and stale tobacco. He was married and had grown children, grandchildren, and great-grandchildren. I wondered what his family thought about him living in Durham full time while they remained in Texas, but I never asked him about it because he was the type of man who wouldn't answer a personal question. He would think it intrusive. So I let Perry talk while I listened.

I interviewed Perry while he was sitting on his favorite couch. I couldn't sit beside him because his girth took up the all the space. I pulled up a metal chair and propped my equipment on my knees. He eyed the tape recorder suspiciously, then folded one of his newspapers and began his tale.

Perry Swain

"I have been on this diet since 1963 and I can tell you all there is to know about it. I was here when there were two Rice Houses: one on Lamont and one on Mangum. You had a choice which Rice House you wanted to go to. I remember when all of the doctors were alive and the Rice House was the place to be. It had a much better clientele back then. Men and women dressed up for meals, there were lively conversations, plays, and entertainment of all kinds. The Rice House was where the rich and famous could hide out without the press hounding them to death.

"Ricers are a lively bunch, and they play a lot of practical jokes because there is nothing much to do in Durham, and eating rice and fruit is boring, and besides, playing jokes is fun. If people get angry over some jokes, then who wants them around anyway? There were more pranks in the old days because people were not as sensitive as they are now, and also, people liked to have fun.

"I was here when Buddy Hackett poured salt in all of the urine bottles. Stood right in the front hall when Kempner kicked him out. I knew of a guy who ate forty hot dogs in one sitting at a Durham Bulls game at the old ballpark. Knew lots of guys who forgot how powerful alcohol was after months on the Rice Diet and found out when they woke up in the drunk tank as guests of the city. But the biggest prank of all was Betty's turkey caper.[22] It is the classic Ricer tale and was Betty's way of saying 'up yours' to Dr. Kempner. She is the only Ricer I ever heard of who stumped the great man.

"Betty was this middle-aged Ricer from New Jersey. She was a short thing, but so fat. Looked like one of those inflatable beach balls. She was wild as a deer, cussed all the time, and kept a fifth of vodka in the back of her Caddy Seville and a .357 Magnum under the front seat. She had a young black man who drove her around, and everyone said they were lovers, but who knows. She had a lot of money. Betty backslid so much on the Diet that Kempner threatened to kick her out for good if she didn't straighten up. Day after day, she would come in and weigh even more than the day before. Kempner accused her of cheating, but she swore up and down that she never ate outside of the Rice House.

"To prove his case and to prevent her from cheating on the Diet, Kempner had her hospitalized for observation. He had the nurses in the hospital keep a close watch on her, monitor all of her food and liquid intake, and keep the door to her room locked at all times. They took the phone from her room so she couldn't call someone to smuggle in food. She was a prisoner. She was in Duke Hospital for three and a half weeks.

"One night, just before Thanksgiving, she found that someone had left the door of her room unlocked. She got out and strolled up and down the halls of the hospital. She didn't care who saw her. The door to the kitchen was left open, and Betty saw the meal carts loaded with trays of turkey waiting to be served the next day. Usually the doors were locked, but for some reason they were open that night. Betty said to herself, 'If it's God's will that that door be open and those turkeys still be there when I come back, then it must be God's will that I have turkey for Thanksgiving.' She walked down the hall and returned to find the turkeys still there. She grabbed the largest one she could find and stuffed it under her hospital robe. Betty weighed herself with the turkey so she could document her heist. She returned to her room, devoured the turkey, and tossed the bones out the window. The next day when Dr. Kempner weighed her, she had put on eleven pounds! Kempner never figured out what happened."

Perry slapped his hands on his knees, and the whole Rice House applauded. While he had been speaking, Ricers and even staff had gathered round to hear the Betty Caper. All of us knew of it already, but due to his age and his place in Ricer culture, Perry had an authority other storytellers lacked. When I left Perry, he was elaborating on the Betty Caper, and other Ricers were adding their accounts.

The second technique vital to success on a diet is the ability to manipulate the body. Many of us have rituals we believe enhance weight loss. Stephen Trehune had an entire series of rituals that he used to lose weight. I met him for an interview in the Regulator Bookshop. Stephen was an actor and lived in Los Angeles. I had seen him on television and in the movies and was a bit awestruck by him. He was very good looking, and many people turned to watch him during the interview. He was in a profession where appearance was critical, so he had to get weight off quickly. If he didn't, he could lose some important roles, and his career would be affected. I found Stephen to be very serious about his weight-loss program. He was dedicated to the Rice Diet.

I was lingering in the magazine section of the shop when I

looked up and saw Stephen through the window. He tapped on the glass and waved, then walked in. I was again struck by how good looking he was. The other customers must have been struck too because they all turned to look at him. Some approached him, but he just smiled and brushed them off. He came over to me and reached up to pull out a magazine. Flipping through the pages, he stopped at one that had his picture with an accompanying article. I took the magazine and skimmed it. Heck, I even bought it.

After a good fifteen minutes of walking around the shop and looking at book titles, we went downstairs to the coffee shop. I set up my equipment while Stephen bought me a coffee and himself a mineral water. He didn't drink coffee because he believed that it aged the body.

I was nervous. It was one thing to talk to him at the Rice House. There he was just another fat guy on the Diet. In the bookshop, he was Stephen Trehune, movie actor. I dropped my notebook, lost my pen, and couldn't plug in my tape recorder because there was no available outlet. I prayed that the batteries would work. All this time, Stephen sat patiently, watching me with a bemused look on his face. He knew I was intimidated by him. Finally I was ready. On cue, in his deep, theater-trained voice he told his story.

Stephen Trehune

"I have been coming to the Rice House for several years and have perfected my personal routine to enhance weight loss. I consider myself a professional dieter. Before I start the Rice Diet, I make a graph of how much weight I intend to lose and by what date. Then I make a bet with my agent to see if I can reach my goal. I place a pretty high bet so the motivation is always there. I start by sitting at the right table. I find one that has successful Ricers who care about their weight loss and don't backslide constantly. I like to sit with old-time Ricers too. I do not like all the questions and life stories of the new people. I find it boring. Sometimes, perhaps after a meal, I will get to know a couple of them, but not during meal time. Then I am there to eat rice and fruit and nothing else.

"I rent a room two miles from the Rice House. That way, I am forced to walk to and from all of my meals. That adds up to twelve miles a day. When I am not eating at the Rice House, I am usually walking to or from it. When I am not walking, I go to the track at Duke and run up and down the steps until I cannot lift my legs anymore. When I get in shape more, I can run up them backwards, but that takes me several weeks of practice. The pain in my calves is unbelievable. I get Percosets to help me through it. I eat rice and fruit, exercise my brains out and zone out with the 'Sets. The lack of sodium in the Diet really helps too, and in a few weeks I look really lean and hungry. Then I leave Durham until I need to come back. I have only lost the bet twice in ten years."

Stephen brought the tips of his fingers together and looked at me. I admired his dedication and said so. He smiled and shook his head. I watched him get up and walk up the stairs. The whole café was watching too.

Jack Talley was another Ricer who had to get his weight off quickly so his career would not suffer. Jack was a professional athlete with a major team. I had seen him at weigh-in at the Rice House. He was so big that he stood out even among a group of very large people. He had absolutely no embarrassment or shame about his weight. He just saw it as a hindrance to his athletic skills. Jack was not fat like the rest of us; rather, he was big, muscular, and bulky. He was funny and liked to tell jokes around the dining room table.

He talked to me right after breakfast, in front of everybody. His tablemates stayed on to hear what he had to say. He signed autographs for a few people and then began talking.

Jack Talley

"There is no way anyone can survive this Diet and not go nuts. You have to be able to cheat a little bit here and there or you might kill somebody over a chicken bone. It could happen. I have seen people, mostly women, get in catfights at the Rice House over portion size. I am not kidding! People take their food allotments very seriously.

Who wouldn't, when all you get is a little handful of rice and some canned fruit in a little tiny bowl? Jesus, this place is awful, but it works. That is why I am here. That is why we are all here.

"I have been coming for three springs in a row, and I know how to work this diet. It is just like anything else. You have to focus on the prize and keep your goal weight in mind. I visualize myself as strong and lean, not big and bulky and sloppy like I usually am. I just keep focusing, but sometimes the need for that taste of good food in my mouth overwhelms me. The first time I was on program when that need came over me, I would end up at the drive-in window at Bojangles and that little backslide would set me back for a week. I would be even more miserable. Now I have found a way to have that taste of good food and still lose weight.

"When the food beats me and I succumb to the need, I go to a restaurant and order five baked potatoes, a big bowl of fruit, and a platter of steamed vegetables. I make sure that the potatoes are plain, without salt or butter, and I can eat what I want and not gain weight. The day after such a feast I may look bigger because I am bound to pick up some unwanted salt somewhere when I eat outside of the Rice House, but I don't gain much weight; maybe eight to ten ounces, but that's it. That is how I manage this Diet."

Jack's way of working the Diet made sense to me and to the other Ricers gathered around the table. We all nodded and mumbled our agreement. Then Jack sprang up, sprinted to the scales, and weighed himself. He was known for weighing several times a day. At morning weigh-in, he would strip down to his boxer shorts. He would probably have removed them if the staff hadn't prevented it.

The final technique, which combines getting along with others and the manipulation of food and the body, is what we call the Celebration: an event that contains elements of fantasy and festivity. Ricer Celebrations are a form of ritual which inverts all the rules of Ricer Culture. These celebrations occur around certain festival dates—Halloween, Super Bowl Sunday, and any weekend when most of the Rice House staff is away on vacation. The hosts of these Celebrations keep the exact dates and locations secret. They pass this information on to chosen Dieters by word of mouth. The ingredients of the Celebrations are the themes of conscious excess, life affirmation, and juxtaposition. A Celebration is the equivalent of the Christmas office party. It is the big blowout where all of the tensions of the Rice Diet are expressed.

I couldn't get a lot of people to agree to give interviews about their involvement in the Celebrations. Their very secrecy and exclusivity prohibited most people from mentioning them.

I brought up the subject of Celebrations at the dinner table one evening and was surprised to find out that another Ricer and I had attended the same party three years earlier. She was a little embarrassed about her attendance at a Celebration but agreed to talk to me if we found a less public place. We walked to my house, and over Red Zinger tea Bonnie recalled the experience.

Bonnie Sherrill

"God, I will never forget my first Celebration. It was something out of a Fellini movie. It was so bizarre and decadent and just plain weird. It was also fascinating because of the excessive consumption of food. It was a delight.

"I had been on program for around six weeks and had lost around twenty-four pounds. I had met some people, and in general was enjoying myself in Durham. One day this young man came over and asked me if I wanted to go to a Super Bowl party. I was flattered that this kid asked me, and thought, 'What the hell? What could it hurt?' I figured his party would consist of some of the younger Ricers having a little bowl of popcorn while watching the Super Bowl. I was curious so I said, 'Okay.' The next day I got a formal invitation in the mail. The invitation was red and the lettering was in gold and quite ornate. I asked some of my friends about it, but nobody knew anything about an upcoming Ricer party.

"The night of the Celebration, I followed the instructions that were enclosed in the invitation and went to an apartment complex near South Square shopping center. When I knocked on the door, the young Ricer kid who had invited me opened it. He was stark naked except for a Dallas Cowboys football helmet. Since I didn't know where to look, I just gazed past him.

"The living room had around twenty-five Ricers in it, in various stages of disarray. I knew most of the folks from the Rice House, but I didn't know them in this way. Some people were getting very affectionate with each other. Some were even putting on a show. There were men and women, and even women and women. You name it—it was going on.

"What really got to me were the buffet tables full of food. You name the food and it was there, all of it forbidden. There was no rice or fruit in sight. The food was elaborate, plentiful, and pleasurable to all of the senses. The host had made ornate displays of food that were beyond anything I had ever seen in L.A., even at the fanciest parties. It was disorienting to see all of that food after the meager fare they serve at the Rice House. My head was spinning. The apartment was wall-to-wall food. Baskets brimming with fresh bread flown in from New York City. Big slabs of butter. Smoked salmon from Scotland, berries from Sweden with clotted cream, cheese of every sort, and pizzas, from thin-crusted to deep-dish. The dessert table was piled high with unimaginable cream cakes, pies, puddings, and other dazzling caloric masterpieces.

"I was mesmerized by the food. People around me were pairing off into couples and retreating into the back bedrooms and out to the hot tub on the deck. People were licking food off each other; the place was wild. I couldn't move. Just looking at the food seemed to cast a spell over me.

"The party went on for hours. By the end of the night there was food splattered over everything: people, walls, carpeting. I am sure that they had to totally redo that whole apartment. When I saw the guests from the party the next morning at weigh-in nobody said a word. It was like the whole evening was a dream, like I had imagined it."

I had been at that same party, but it wasn't strange that Bonnie and I didn't recognize each other. That night had seemed bizarre to me as well. Several people were in costume, and many of them I did not recognize. The everyday rules of living seemed reversed. The dominant personalities were subdued, and the quiet ones were boisterous. The boundaries of relationships were gone, too.

People that I had seen together for weeks at the Rice House showed up with their regular partners but left with someone else. I had gone with one man I knew, but he vanished and I wound up with a bunch of people that I had never met. Everything was very loose and easy, except for the food.

The food I remember vividly. It was fantastic to look at. Every forbidden food was there. Funny, but the only thing I really wanted was vegetables. I had eaten rice and fruit for so long that I could not stand the taste of anything sweet. I wanted vegetables and bread. I gained four pounds from that one celebration, and it took me two weeks to get it off. That was the last party I attended for many months.

Many of us view dieting as an occupation. I have been doing it as long as I remember, so eating less and exercising more to lose weight is a way of life. Unfortunately, as with an occupation, I diet forty hours a week and take the weekends and holidays off. That way, I rationalize to myself, I can separate myself from the rest of the world's disorderly eating behavior by dieting during the week. I can rejoin the world on weekends and pretend I am normal, like everyone else. Besides, I have found that people really resent dieters. When I am invited to dinner parties and I eat only a third of my food, the host and even the guests keep quizzing me about dieting. Their remarks range from, "Are you still dieting?" to "Obviously dieting doesn't work for you, so you might as well eat and enjoy yourself." It is much easier to eat what is put in front me.

I wish I could say that dieting this way has lessened the tension I have around food. Unfortunately, it has not. Food still makes me nervous, and if I could totally eliminate my exposure to diet-busting food, it would be easier to lose weight. Those Ricers who see the Diet as a form of worship do this, and they really lose a lot of weight and keep it off longer than those of us who see dieting as an occupation. I just can't maintain that zeal for dieting. I never converted to the Rice Diet, I merely followed it. Yet, even though I never got near my goal weight, I lost enough to experience the last step of the Dieter's experience at the Rice House—the Redemption stage.

eleven

Redemption

The Redemption stage is where the affirmation of the Rice Diet blooms. It is the last stage of the Dieting experience. At this point, we get the payoff for all those months of staying in Durham on the program. Even though we may not have attained the grail of goal weight, we have lost a significant amount of weight, and a new life begins. Those who do reach goal rarely maintain it, but the power of it is strong and motivates all of us to try to reach this stage.

Those of us who had lost a great deal of weight and were preparing to leave the Rice House and reenter the dominant culture would often sit on the front porch after supper and speculate on our new lives. It reminded me of summers at camp, where campmates sit around the fire and dream out loud about the future. In Durham, we convinced ourselves that we would never regain any weight. We were now too evolved for that. Instead we would continue the work on our bodies, minds, and souls that we had begun here. None of us would go back to life before the Rice Diet.

Redemption brings with it opportunity, joy, power, and satisfaction beyond one's expectations. It also brings disorientation, stagnation, sadness, and regret. Weight loss changes everything about a person—about a life.

Many of us who lose a lot of weight feel born again, and this time into the right body. Abby Felcher felt that her life began again once she reached her goal weight. Abby and some of our friends joined me for a evening at my house. Abby was celebrating because she was almost to goal weight (again) and would be going home a thin woman. Another friend was getting married, and a new friend was celebrating a twenty-pound loss. For the occasion, I offered a variety of flavored rice crackers, plain, unsalted, air-popped popcorn, seltzer water, and a bottle of California champagne. It was only enough for each of us to get a sip, so I didn't think we would consume very many calories. After half an hour of socializing, people found places to sit, and Abby began talking about becoming thin.

Abby Felcher

"When I did it, when I finally got on that scale and it said 115 pounds and the whole room erupted in applause, I felt such a shift inside me that I thought I was going to fall off the scale. All of my life I had planned that moment, worked for it, postponed it, turned my back on it, and tried finally to do it—to lose all of my weight. When I reached goal I felt just like Sleeping Beauty being kissed by Prince Charming. All of my life I had been asleep. Oh, I lived it, time passed, I had joys and sorrows, but I really didn't feel as if I was the main lead in my own life. When I hit goal weight I woke up. I let go of the past; even more than that, I didn't even recognize my own past. It was like somebody else had lived that life. I looked in the mirror and didn't recognize myself.

"I was somebody different, somebody new."

Abby finished talking and reached for her wine glass. She was beaming with happiness. The rest of us looked around at each other and thought the same thing. Would we ever feel that way? Would we get to goal?

After the party, Abby stayed to help me tidy up. She was almost giddy with excitement about returning home thin, but sad to leave Durham. We promised to keep in touch and to visit each other often. I was tearful at seeing Abby leave. She was my close friend, my guide to diet culture, and my mentor in many ways. She told me to keep doing it, keep losing weight. She got in her car and drove home that night.

Kae Heiman, a thirty-year-old playwright, had a similar born-again experience. Kae had seesawed between thinness and obesity all of her life. I met her when I returned to the Rice House to lose more weight and collect more stories. She was very thin when I met her, and I couldn't imagine her ever being fat. She had a wicked sense of humor and would often tell me funny stories about fellow Ricers. I was careful of what I said around her because I would hear something I told her repeated later, and her version of my story always had unusual and risqué twists. Kae's interests were in a good story rather than the facts.

We met at an bar in Durham. I had thought that I had been in every bar, restaurant, and coffee shop in the Triangle area, but this was a surprise. Leave it to Kae to know of the most obscure, yet interesting, spot. Kae was like that, an insider.

She was smoking when I entered the dark bar. When I got closer, I saw that it was a hand-rolled, filterless cigarette. Kae explained to me that she enjoyed her smokes straight up, without the protective barrier of a filter. I looked down to see if she was drinking her water straight up too. Kae refrained from all alcohol. She felt it was bad for her weight. Cigarettes, on the other hand, helped her maintain her waif-like figure.

I heaved myself up into the high barstool as gracefully as possible and looked hard in her face. Kae said she was somewhere in her thirties, but it was rumored that she was more like fifty. The cigarettes and constant weight cycling should have taken their toll, yet she looked wonderful. I asked her what it was like to get there, to reach goal weight and she responded.

Kae Heiman

"Reaching goal weight was a renaissance. My life began again, and this time it was the right life for me: a thin one. How did 110 pounds feel? It just felt natural. I only stayed at that weight for about two weeks, but it was worth it. For the first time, everything in my life was right. Being thin is just fabulous. You feel great and the world treats you better. The thing that gets me is how easy it is to get along in the world when you are thin. As a fat person, I was constantly trying to squeeze myself in a world full of tight spaces, and there was this cloud over my head reminding me that I was fat. Life is hard when you are fat. The world is meant for small people: airplane seats, movie seats, dressing rooms, desks at school, furniture, and especially clothes. When I was fat, everything in the world shouted at me that I did not fit; I was too big.

"People just looked right past me when I was fat. I can never understand it, but the thinner I am, the more visible I become. It is a strange sensation. People are easier to deal with because they see me as an equal instead of this subhuman life form. They also view me as competent and intelligent. I don't have to prove myself, I don't have to do anything but stay thin, and of course, never tell people that I was ever fat. The people who knew me before I can't do anything about, but when I meet new people, I never tell them that I was once morbidly obese. Dr. Kempner told me that there is as much prejudice against the formerly fat as there is against the currently fat. People are so repulsed by weight that they damn you if you have ever been fat. A guy at the Rice House told me to never, under any circumstance, tell any guy that I was ever fat. He told me that at the most, I could say that I had lost forty pounds. You see, thin people think anyone who is over forty pounds overweight is huge, monstrous. To be on the safe side I never mention weight to anyone.

"Staying thin is the hardest part of my life because the entire United States, and perhaps the whole Western world, is on a binge. Everything and everyone is telling us to eat. It was so hard to go out to dinner with people after I got to goal weight, especially people who had known me fat. I was self-conscious and very much aware that others were looking at my food choices and intake. I knew they were silently judging me. It was difficult to go home thin after being at the Rice House. For the first couple of weeks, everyone was cheering me on and saying congratulations, but after the initial joy of it all, reality set in and the weight loss was no big deal anymore. It is still a big deal to me, but not to my friends and family. I know that they are saying to themselves stuff like, 'She'll never keep it off, she'll gain it all back.' That is the only hard part I have encountered with getting thin; nobody thinks I can maintain my weight loss, nobody. I guess they are right in that assumption. I have been really thin before, but gained it all back. To me, thin is like visiting a foreign country. I plan about it, read about it, finally get there and take a lot of pictures to prove to myself that I have actually been to that thin place, but I always return home to fat. Fat is the usual, the familiar to me. It is where I live."

I knew exactly what Kae meant. Even though I wasn't thin, I think about it as a destination. Not something I will be, but someplace I will reach. I am on the road to thinness. I may never get there, but if I do, I will take a lot of pictures.

Susan Tucker was born again too. I knew Susan when she began at the Rice House and saw her lose all the way to goal weight. It was an amazing transformation. I had lost a lot of weight too and sometimes even considered myself a normal size. Susan assured me that I was not thin or even within the range of acceptable weight. I was disappointed to hear her say it, but it didn't hurt me because I had told myself the same thing many times. She just confirmed my suspicions.

I met Susan at Northgate Mall. She was there at the tailor shop having her clothes cut down to fit her tiny size. While I waited in the food court, I watched shoppers pass by. Most appeared overweight, tired, and in a hurry. Out of the crowd came Susan, tall, thin, and elegant in tailored jeans and a tight cashmere sweater. People turned as she walked by.

She slid into the plastic molded seat at the table, plopped her packages on the dirty floor, and opened the bottle of mineral water she always carried with her. After downing half of it, she recapped the bottle and put it back in her bag. I waited until she was settled and asked her to tell me what it was like being thin.

Susan Tucker

"Being thin makes all the difference in the world. It is like having a new life. I was fat off and on throughout most of my life and fat all of my adult life, so I grew up in a certain way. I knew it wasn't a good way to grow up. I could look around me and see that society rewarded thin people and punished the fat. I had a crappy life, let's face it. I was never the lead in a play in high school; I was the prop lady. I wasn't the starring ballerina in dance class when I was a child, but part of the scenery. I was always the last one picked for everything. Even my parents didn't value me as much as they did my thin siblings. The strange thing about my life and its limitations is I just accepted it as the way things were. I didn't question my role or others' expectations of me. I felt that something was wrong, and I knew it was my weight, but it wasn't until I got to goal weight that I realized the extent of my marginalization.

"My redemption, or new life, started before I even reached goal weight, but not until I dropped under 140 pounds. Anything above that and you are still fat. You may not think of yourself as fat, and people may tell you that you look fine, but they're lying. It wasn't until I got below 140 that life just burst open. Opportunities, jobs, happiness, success, good health, even love just came to me overnight. It was as though fate said, 'Okay, your turn.' Thinness means everything is possible. I am never going back to fat."

She reached for her water, took another gulp, and then was on her way. There were clothes to buy, errands to run, and lovers to meet. Her whole life was waiting for her now that she was thin, and she had to be on her way. She grabbed her packages and rushed out of the food court. Again, people turned to look at her. I sat at the table a few moments longer, then gathered my things and walked back to the Rice House.

Mark Alexander, a native of New York City, got a new life when he lost his weight, too. I had known Mark off and on during his stays in Durham, and I had seen him in his various stages of weight loss. He used to look like a cuddly panda bear with round soft cheeks and dreamy eyes. Now he looked like a bird of prey, an eagle or a hawk. He was tall with sharp features and had a habit of always looking around as if he was afraid that someone was sneaking up on him.

I met Mark at Shoney's for coffee. Shoney's used to be his favorite backsliding site because of their chocolate fudge cake. Now Mark went there for decaffeinated coffee. We chatted for an hour. The waitress often returned to refill our coffee cups. I knew refills at Shoney's were free, and Mark liked that. I had heard from others at the Rice House that he was very cheap and wouldn't pick up the tab for anyone, not even himself. He was the forty-year-old owner of several multimedia companies worldwide and could probably have bought out the whole Shoney's chain if he'd wanted to.

After his third refill of coffee and water, Mark finally got to the point. He flipped his long legs up on the booth and stretched out. He looked like he might take a nap. Instead he began his tale.

Mark Alexander

"Thinness brings new life. That bullshit that you are still you when you are fat or thin, that the real you is unchanged, is total crap. The world loves you thin and hates you fat. Let's face it, when you are fat you look at another fat guy on the street and you have this silent communication going on. You nod to each other and it's understood. You've recognized your own kind. When you get thin, you see the same guy on the street and glance away and say to yourself, 'What a slob. How disgusting.' That's what I do now. When I see someone fat, I think, 'What a total loser. Glad I am not that guy.' It's weird that I feel this way now because before, when I was fat, I was the champion of fat people. I would argue about discrimination and fat people's rights, but now that I am thin, I don't give a shit about fat people. Fuck 'em. I am not one of them anymore. I am on the other side. I am thin.

"I feel so powerful thin, like I can do anything. And the way people respond to me is unbelievable. Everyone is eager to please me, whereas before they just tried to stay away from me or looked past me. I have people calling me up offering me deals, where before they wouldn't even answer my phone calls. Women are throwing themselves at me. It is definitely because of the weight, because I was rich before, but I was fat. Even my old girlfriend from college called me up and said, 'Oh Mark, Mark, I hear you have changed. Can we get together?' No, we cannot get together. I did meet up with her for one night, and she was all over me. Before, when I was morbidly obese, I had to beg her for sex, and now she wants to give me a blow job in the car—and all because I lost a hundred pounds?

"I met this one girl at the Rice House who was about nineteen years old and really, really fat. She got down to 110 pounds. She decided to go home and screw with everyone that treated her bad. She was into this revenge thing. She did go home looking fantastic, like a model. When she got to goal she bought herself a red leather minidress with laces up the front. She looked good in that dress. Walked around Durham in these high-heeled boots. I will never forget it. Last time I heard from her she had credited herself with breaking up three marriages so far. That girl was on a mission. I don't have any kind of mission other than to enjoy my new and improved life, and to stay thin forever."

Mark signaled the waitress and asked for the bill. I was surprised. Maybe the rumors about him weren't true. Perhaps he wasn't so cheap. When the waitress started to hand him the slip, he pointed to me. I took it, paid the two dollars, and left another two for the tip. I walked Mark to his car, a sporty little two-seater with a set of golf clubs sticking out the back, and watched as he drove off.

Joyce Calanero was born again at goal weight and, like others I have interviewed, found the world a much more hospitable place for a thin person. I met her at the Rice House for the interview because Joyce liked to limit her exposure to forbidden food. She felt safe at the Rice House.

Joyce loved being thin and was very proud of her weight loss, but she also felt disappointed in a world that was so shallow. When she was fat, she hoped that people looked beyond her weight to her personality, but the world only measured her by her weight, not by her accomplishments.

We met after lunch. A few Ricers hung around to see what was going on. Some wondered out loud why a thin person was eating at the Rice House at all. Joyce looked at me, and I knew what she was thinking. She was thin now, and some people resented her.

They judged her by her weight, and now it was too low. Before her weight loss, the world had said she was too fat. There was no middle ground. As the waitstaff cleared away the empty plates, I asked Joyce how she felts now that she was at goal weight. What was it like living thin? Joyce looked at her hands and began to speak.

Joyce Calanero

"The world worships you when you are thin. Life is easy thin. You don't have to do anything, and you get rewarded for it. I will tell you a true story. I was going to be at the Rice House for a long time. I had over a hundred pounds to lose to get to goal weight, and I was determined to do it. I decided that if things were going well and I was losing weight at an appropriate speed after a few months on program, I would get a job—not a demanding job that would cut into my walking and exercise time, but some little job, a few afternoons a week.

"I saw an ad in the newspaper classifieds for a part-time secretary position at the University of North Carolina at Chapel Hill. It was for some study on gifted children they were doing. That was just the kind of job I was looking for. I weighed maybe 200 pounds at the time. I had lost approximately seventy-five pounds. I got dressed in business attire: basic black suit from Saks Fifth Avenue, white blouse, dark stockings, classic pumps and a subdued handbag. Had my hair, makeup, and nails done. Polished up my résumé, which was already nearly perfect. I had taught for fifteen years at a well-known prep school. I knew how to type, use a computer, and everything else they wanted.

"The moment I walked in the office the receptionist just assumed I was there for the secretary job, which of course, I was. There were a bunch of other people there applying for all sorts of jobs, so I could have been there for any position, but she just thought I 'looked' secretarial. I got the message, which was: fat people deserve low-paying clerical and staff jobs. The interview went well, but I didn't get the job. Months later I saw that the same people were advertising for another secretary. I was still looking for a job so I went again. This time I weighed around 140 pounds.

Again, I wore appropriate business attire, but this time the same receptionist took one look at me and assumed I was there for the director's job. She put me in an office by myself, brought me coffee and something to read, and basically waited on me. I gave her a copy of my résumé, and she came back later with the outgoing director. Everyone was thrilled with me and my credentials. When I told them that I was there for the secretarial position, they just blinked. They couldn't believe it. The moral of this story is that fat means failure, thin means success."

Joyce pushed back her chair. The few Ricers that were still hanging around nodded in agreement. Most people in the room had been both fat and thin, and all of us knew that being thin meant having an easier time of it. I left Joyce at the table. I had a meeting to attend. On the drive to Chapel Hill I tried to imagine what it would be like for me to be that thin. Would I get everything I ever wanted and more? Does everyone who gets thin have an better life?

Sloane Dixon had a startling Redemption experience. Her story was well known around the Rice House. I'd asked her for an interview months before because she was a woman who had the made the most dramatic changes in herself. She got to goal weight, had extensive plastic surgery, got married, divorced, remarried, divorced again, and even changed her first name. I admired her because she had the guts to do it, to change everything and become the person she always dreamed she could be.

She came to my house for the interview and brought me a present—a beautiful white orchid plant. I was taken aback by such a gesture. I didn't know her that well and it was an expensive gift. I thanked her for her thoughtfulness and began to set up. Sloane walked to the dining room and selected one of the chairs. She sat down on the very edge of it with her athletic legs curved to the side. She looked like she was sitting for a portrait. I unplugged my tape recorder, picked up my notebooks and hauled everything to the dining room. I reached down to find an outlet, and Sloane started talking.

Sloane Dixon

"I have been fat all of my life. My first memory is of my mother yelling at me because I was eating too much. I was never allowed to eat in my house, because my parents were freaks about weight gain. They hated the obese, and as fate would have it, they had obese kids: three of them. I got married when I was right out of high school, and I was fat too. I got fatter with each child, but it was okay because it was expected that I would just get fatter and fatter. Of course, my doctor and family nagged me constantly about my weight, but they knew it would never change; I would never lose weight. My husband nagged me too, but there was this unspoken agreement between us that he would tolerate my excess weight as long as I was not too demanding and as long as I didn't ask too much of him or of our marriage. We went on like that for years. I had very low expectations of marriage and of life in general.

"I was the fat one, and, like the sick one in the family, I got special treatment. Really, being fat has some sort of special power: all the attention is negative, but it still has power. Special accommodations had to be made for me because I was fat. I couldn't participate in athletic or some social activities. I couldn't be expected to put on a bathing suit and go to the beach, play tennis or golf, or do any other kind of sport. Parties and other gatherings were out of the question because everyone felt uncomfortable about me, especially my husband and children. They were embarrassed because I was so fat, but they were used to it. My husband ran interference with the world to protect me, and I, in turn, provided the nurturing maternal role that seemed to satisfy him on some deep, unexamined level. I guess we both benefited from it.

"When I lost all of my weight, it was as though I was risen up from the dead. I felt like I was surfacing. Really, I guess I had been drowning for years and didn't even realize it. When I got to goal weight, all hell broke loose. I wanted everything that had been denied me when I was fat. All those lost years, all those lost opportunities—I wanted it all back so I could do it over again, and this time do it right. It was so jarring to be thin. I was so bored. People are boring when you get thin, boring and stupid. I didn't think they were when I was fat. Then, I wanted to be just like those people. Now, I don't have time for people I don't like. I can't stand boring people. I am not satisfied with flopping down on the couch in front of the tube with three Domino's pizzas lined up on the floor like the old days. I can't stand television. It's boring. I can't waste time anymore.

"When I got thin, the first thing I did was go back to school and get my college degree. I didn't care if I got a diploma: I just wanted young, interesting, and energetic people around me. I wanted social stimulation. I wanted fun.

"Two years after goal weight, I had plastic surgery, and I have never regretted it. I went to Brazil to have the surgery, then I went to California for the recovery time. While there I had a total makeover: hair, clothes, jewelry. My family couldn't stand it. They wanted the old me back, but the old me was dead and gone. I felt like someone who had been let out of prison after being condemned to a life sentence. My husband filed for divorce and moved out. My children are stunned by me. They used to be embarrassed because I was so fat; now they are mad because I look so good. I lost weight, lost my husband and even my children, but it is worth it. I found myself."

Sloane finished her story and drummed her fingers on the table. I looked at her hands—manicured nails, pristine skin without a blemish—and wondered if she'd had plastic surgery on them, even though I wasn't sure if that was possible. Sloane looked like a living Barbie doll and was beautiful in a toy-like way. Close up, I found her rather frightening. My thoughts must have showed on my face, because Sloane sniggered and pulled up the sleeve of her silk blouse to show me her surgery scar. Her upper arm was mottled and puckered, and the stitching looked like Frankenstein's. Instead of being horrified, I was relieved. At least she was human. At least she was imperfect. She ran her pretty fingers up and down the jagged scar and we both laughed out loud. I walked her to the door and thanked her again for the flower. She adjusted her sleeve and left.

Sam Pratto's family didn't like him thin either. Like Sloane's family, Sam's wife and children didn't know what to do with an ex-fatty. I met Sam at the Rice House for his interview. I had known Sam for several years. He dated a friend of mine, and I knew a lot about him from her. Sam was a retired real estate investor from Palm Springs, California. He was divorced with grown children and grandchildren. Sam has kept his weight off and had plastic surgery to remove the excess skin from his stomach.

I interviewed Sam in the clay room of the Durham Arts Council building. Sam had taken up pottery while on the Diet. He found it soothing and time-consuming. He had gotten some clay for me and watched as I attacked it. After a few moments, he came over and showed me how it was done. I decided to make a platter. How hard could that be? A platter was easy and useful. Sam didn't have a plan in mind for his clay. He just liked working with it.

I checked the batteries in my tape recorder and pressed the start button. I nodded to Sam to begin, and as he punched the clay like bread dough he started talking.

Sam Pratto

"I was always the fat boy. I was fat when my wife married me. She called me her teddy bear, and she liked the bigness of me. She said she liked a hefty man. I went on the Rice Diet because my doctors told me to. I was so sick with multiple diseases, and if I hadn't lost weight I would have died. I stayed at the Rice House until I got to goal. It took me two years to do it, but I did and I have never regretted it. I can do things that normal people take for granted: breathe without pain, sit in a chair comfortably, fit behind the wheel of a car, and just live. I love being thin.

"I thought everyone would be thrilled that I got to goal weight. After all, my family has been telling me for years to lose weight and I finally did it. My family was *not* thrilled, but instead downright hostile. I had seen my wife often over the two years I was on program, so it wasn't such a shock for her to see me thin. She had been a witness to the process. She was happy for me when I reached goal because she knew that it was a big milestone for me, but you could tell she was unnerved by it. I asked her what was wrong and she assured me that nothing was wrong and everything was fine. When I moved back home, you could feel the hostility in the air. My wife didn't like to prepare special Ricer meals for me and couldn't understand why I had to have plain food without salt. She thought I should be able to eat what other people ate, but not eat as much of it. I can't do that. Once I get the taste of salt in my mouth, I just want more of it, more food.

"Nothing was the same after I reached goal. Everyone acted like they didn't know me, and I guess they didn't. I left this huge fat guy who could barely move off the sofa, and I came back a healthy, thin man full of pep. I wanted to run around and have fun, and all of my friends were old and sick and waiting for the grave. My wife couldn't stand me. She wanted the old fat me back—her old cushy teddy bear—but that me was gone for good. I wanted to have sex all the time now that I could, and she said that part of her life was behind her. My kids were angry at me all the time because they said I wasn't acting my age. They just didn't get it. I had a new lease on life, and nobody wanted me to take it. I guess they were all waiting for me to die, and I lived."

He stopped talking and backed away from the table to observe his work. I looked over to see what he had created—a large object that looked like a six-legged horse. He worked with clay for therapy, not for art. I was pretty proud of my work; the platter looked good. I painted it tan and turquoise for a Southwestern feel. Sam said we could leave our stuff on a nearby shelf and the staff would put it in the kiln for us. A week later I dropped by the Arts Council to pick up my platter. Unfortunately, it had broken during the heating process. I gathered the shattered pieces and put them in my tote bag. Later, I lined the bottom of a pot with them and planted the orchid Sloane had given me.

Sylvia Moffitt loved her weight loss, but not the baggy body left behind. I met Sylvia in my first month at the Rice House, and I loved her stories about Ricer lore. She was a great talker and always had an audience around her. She had a lot of friends, but I never saw her outside the Rice House. I assume she never ate outside it. I interviewed her right at the dining room table after lunch. I knew Sylvia was the owner of a recording company and lived in California. I learned from others that she was divorced and had no children.

I was sitting in the parlor and waved to Sylvia as she walked in. She nodded but went off to weigh herself in another room. Like many dieters, she often weighed, sometimes three or four times a day. I hated to weigh. It depressed rather than inspired me. I guess for Sylvia, the scale was the monitor.

After weighing, she came in and plopped down beside me on the couch. Squeezing my hand, she started chattering about her day. I just smiled and let her go on. Quietly readying my equipment, I waited for a break in Sylvia's monologue. Finally, she took a deep breath and told her story.

Sylvia Moffitt

"I never got to goal weight, but I got close enough that I could actually see the numbers on the scale. I lost 175 pounds on the Rice Diet the first time I ever went on it. That was in 1988, and I never let my weight gain get up to more than seven or eight pounds before I do something about it. I come back to Durham at least four times a year to maintain my weight loss. I have gained thirty pounds from my first big loss, but I have held the line at that.

"I was so amazed when I hit goal that I really didn't know how to act. I didn't know how to exist without dealing with an excess of weight. It was weird to be thin after so many years of being fat. My body didn't know how to react either. I was so clumsy. I had to take dance classes and physical therapy sessions to learn how to move my body. Right after I got to goal, I sprained my ankle. I was so used to heaving three hundred pounds around that I would literally fly out of a chair. You know how when you are fat and you sit on a low couch or chair you have to position yourself, brace yourself so you don't sink too far down and can eventually get out without too much struggle? Well, I was used to doing that, and then after I lost weight, I didn't have to use that much force. You would think that my body would have adjusted through the months of weight loss to my thinner self, but that didn't happen. The physical therapist told me that the reason I kept injuring myself was because my ligaments had been so stretched for so long that they were just too loose for my joints. I had to go to therapy for months and do all of these exercises to get my ligaments back into shape. Now I can move like a thin person because I guess I am one.

"I thought my skin would go back into place and I wouldn't have to have any kind of surgery. I know of several women at the Rice House who had had some body work done and they look terrible: all that scarring and puckering. The plastic surgeon told me that the purpose of plastic surgery is to make you look better clothed, not naked. I don't get that. I want to look great naked or clothed. I thought sure I would, too, because I exercised faithfully, slathered expensive skin-firming creams all over me and drenched my thighs in Clarins thigh-firming cream. I had deep tissue massage and everything else they tell you will help. Yet when I lost weight my body looked like something moved out.

"My skin is like fabric: it drapes, pulls, even tears. I bruise and hurt myself more easily than I did fat. I lift up my arm and I have this swing of flesh that follows a few moments later. I hate it. I have done triceps exercises for years to no avail. The doctor says I have great muscle tone. Unfortunately, it's covered by a blanket of loose flesh. I can always tell if someone has lost a hundred pounds or more. Put me in any Loemann's dressing room and I can pick out the ex-fatties. Women who have lost a hundred pounds have battle scars: a little triangle of flesh right above the navel, diagonal fold lines across the upper thighs and droopy knees. The body remembers."

Sylvia finished her story and popped her blouse open for me to see the results of her successful weight loss. Nobody at the Rice House even looked up. They were used to seeing near-naked people, usually on the scale. People took off everything possible for weigh-in. I looked at Sylvia's stomach and found the telltale triangle of loose skin. Her upper arms looked deflated and reminded me of chicken wings. She had a couple of empty rolls of skin that hung on her upper stomach. Her breasts, however, were firm, high, and round as grapefruits. They looked misplaced on her body, like some mad scientist had put them on the wrong torso. I knew they were not real. Everyone at the Rice House knew too.

Sylvia was known to flash them around at the dinner table, proud of her new breasts. As I sat there staring at them, I wondered what archaeologists would think, hundreds of years from now, when they dig up the bodies of Durham and wonder at the sight of the withered, decayed bones of a lost tribe topped by two hard balloons of silicone. Would they think the silicone balls were a type of deformity or objects of worship? History will judge.

Elizabeth Chiesa was proud of her weight loss, but disgusted by her sagging skin. I met Elizabeth at a clothes swap that a group of Ricers had put together. The clothes swap was a good idea because we lose weight so fast on the Diet that we can't afford to buy new clothes to keep up with our changing selves. We take our old fat clothes and exchange them for smaller ones. I was thrilled when I could dump my size eighteens and sixteens and put on smaller, cuter clothes. I was also delighted that I got some quality clothes. To this day, my mother still wears a sweatsuit that I picked up at a clothes swap a decade ago.

Elizabeth was changing clothes in a fellow Ricer's living room during a swap, and she caught me glancing at her body. I was fascinated and repelled by her loose skin and was worried that I would have the same problem. Elizabeth was very honest about her body and spoke candidly. I interviewed her at her apartment in Durham, which was filled with photos of her family. She had a warm and friendly place done in soft pastels. It looked like something that belonged in California or Florida or some place at the beach. I sat down in a rattan chair, and Elizabeth brought us some mineral water and fresh peaches. As I reached over for a peach, Elizabeth placed her hand over mine and spoke.

Elizabeth Chiesa

"I am so thankful to be thin. Losing weight has changed my life in every way possible, and I am grateful for all of the wonderful things that have happened to me. The only area of my life that really disappoints me is my body. It is always my body. When I was fat, I hated my body because of the weight. Now that I am thin, I hate my body because it was once fat, if that makes sense.

"My body looks like it is morphed between a thin person and a fat person: part of me still has the remains of a fat person, and part of me looks skinny. I am almost as limited now as I was when I was fat. I still don't wear a bathing suit, or shorts, or skirts. My legs are too lumpy. I lost the weight, but my skin is baggy and the muscles underneath bunch up in little clots. That is my muscle buildup. I can't help that. I always did have very muscular legs. My breasts, what's left of them, look long and thin, like bananas. The skin on my stomach is droopy, but not enough to have a tuck. My feet and hands seem huge to me. I guess my body was so big that my feet and hands just looked small, but really, I have gone up two sizes in shoes since I lost weight. My face looks very angled and sharp. I never realized I had such a long nose until I lost weight. I look older than I am. I look haggard. My rear end flattened out like an ironing board. I used to have a high-looking ass, but now it is all droopy. I do squats all the time, but they don't do any good.

"People who really look at me can tell I have lost a lot of weight. When I reached goal, I went to Glamour Shots to have a makeover, and the man who did my makeup asked me point-blank how much weight I had lost. He knew I had lost over ninety pounds. He said he can always tell by the collarbones. I was so self-conscious after the session that I would wear turtlenecks so people couldn't tell that I had been fat. It is horrible how weight still plagues me.

"The thing that disappoints me most about my weight loss is now I am ordinary. Before, I had a lot of attention. Most of it was rude, and I knew that I looked like a freak, but at least I looked different; I was special. Now I look like everyone else. You can go to any mall in America and see a hundred women who look just like me. I guess that I had thought that when I got thin, I would look like a movie star. I thought I would look like Kathleen Turner in *Body Heat*. I really did believe that. Now, I don't look like anybody, not even myself."

Elizabeth looked confused and went off to the kitchen to get more water. I was flabbergasted. What's the good in losing a ton of weight if you still feel uncomfortable in your body? Would it never end? Were we doomed to be disappointed by our bodies and our lives? Would the ghost of fat always haunt us? Elizabeth came back with new bottles of water and refilled our glasses. I felt uncomfortable and had no idea what to say. She smiled and tried to make conversation, but neither one of us said much. I thanked her for her time and literally backed out of the room. In my car, I studied my face and neck in the rear-view mirror. When I got thin, would my skin hold up? Would it remain elastic and resilient or succumb to weight loss and time?

My story is similar to those of my informants and to that of every Ricer who has lost a lot of weight. I was thrilled when my name went up on the Century Board at the Rice House. People I had known for a long time came up and congratulated me, and the staff was very proud. New Ricers just wanted to know how long it had taken me to lose the weight. They used me as a gauge to figure out how long it would take them to get their weight off. I was surprised to find that I was an example to others struggling with the Diet.

The Dieting community understood my weight loss, and old Ricers that I had never met while on program would stop me on the street to cheer me on. I felt like I was walking on air, and that there was nothing that I couldn't do. I felt beautiful and powerful. To the nondieting world, though, I was now average. I wasn't massively obese, nor was I stylishly thin. I was just plain average. I guessed that Susan Tucker was right when she said that I had to get below 140 pounds for it to count, for people to take notice.

I was disappointed by the reaction of the general population. Even the nurse at the Rice House told me, "You may think you are thin, but to the rest of the world you are still chubby." I hate the words chubby and plump because, to me, they refer to a holding pattern of weight. I like stark contrasts. I like words like fat or thin, obese or slim. They have meaning. They take a stand. Chubby and plump mean you are between opposites.

I assured myself that since the general nondieting population didn't know me or my history, their reaction didn't count for much. I knew that my family, unlike those families of some of the Ricers I interviewed, would be delighted and amazed at my weight loss. When I lost a hundred pounds on the Rice Diet, I decided that I would have an official unveiling. My family was to meet at my sister's house in Maplewood, New Jersey, for Christmas. No one outside the Rice House had seen me since my tremendous weight loss. I searched for the perfect dress, a style I had always wanted to wear. I bought a black turtleneck sweater-knit dress that fit me like a glove. I bought a pair of black stiletto heels to go with it. I borrowed a long black leather coat from a fellow Ricer, and had my hair done up in a French twist. I had my makeup and nails done professionally and borrowed a pair of diamond earrings for the occasion. The whole Rice House got into the production of creating the perfect me as a surprise for my family and friends.

The day of my flight north I prepared as if I were going on the ultimate date. It took me several hours to get ready, and when I showed up at the Rice House for my last meal there, people took pictures, and I felt like Cinderella on her way to the ball. As I boarded the plane at the Raleigh-Durham airport I told just about everyone of my adventure. My fellow passengers were as excited as I was. When the plane landed in Newark, I could barely contain my excitement.

My expectations crumbled when there was nobody there to meet me. Finally, a friend of my sister's showed up and drove me to my sister's house. The friend thought I looked nice, but she didn't know me from Adam so what difference did it make? Nobody was at the house when I arrived. My parents and sister showed up later. Not one word was said about my weight loss. Instead they asked if I had had a pleasant flight, how long would I be I staying, and wasn't the weather awful? My mother and father sat glued to the TV most of the time and ate M&Ms out of a big bowl on the coffee table. I asked them directly what they thought of my weight loss. My father shrugged and stated that I still had a ways to go. Finally, late that evening, as I was brushing my teeth in the bathroom, my sister commented on my weight loss indirectly. I was standing at the sink in my bra and panties and she said, "Wow. I can see a rib or two." That was it. After a very depressing holiday, I returned to Durham. My life, despite my family's passive reaction, changed dramatically.

After losing a hundred pounds, I was born again into a much

happier world. Opportunities and experiences that had been closed to me opened up. I got job offers galore. Headhunters called me for a change. I got into graduate school, dated people I had only read about in the newspapers. Old friends I had forgotten called me. A guy I had met one night in Santa Cruz, California four years earlier tracked me down in Durham because he'd heard from a friend that I had lost a lot of weight.

Nothing about me was the same. My family knew it. The moment they saw me that Christmas in New Jersey they knew that I would never be the emotional buffer I was raised to be. My friends knew it. No more would I be their secret diet cheater or meet them in out-of-the-way restaurants to eat forbidden food. No more would I listen to their litany of complaints about their jobs, husband, or children. I was done with all that.

I arranged to meet my old non-Ricer boyfriend in New York on New Year's Eve. I had planned what I thought would be a spectacular weekend. He had seen me once while I was on the Rice Diet and that was right after I started the program. I was so nervous and hungry and longing just for the way it used to be between us. When I got off the plane I went directly to the lounge and ordered a drink. It was the first taste of alcohol I'd had in a year. While I was at it, I had a couple of shooters on the side. By the time my boyfriend's plane arrived, I was quite drunk. He was stunned to see me. He'd never seen me that thin or that intoxicated before. We drove into the city in silence.

My boyfriend, like my parents, was astounded by my weight loss and didn't know how to react. I just sat in the car and got more depressed. I spent the weekend drinking myself into oblivion. I could restrain my eating, but I couldn't restrain my drinking. Instead of craving food, I craved alcohol, or rather, that kick you get from drinking it. I wanted to drink and drink until I felt that click in my head. I wanted to drink until I was floating and feeling no pain—the same feeling I used to get from eating potato chips and M&Ms when I was a child—but food could no longer play that role for me. I knew I was just replacing one addiction with another. I quit drinking that weekend. I returned to Durham more determined than ever to attain goal weight.

twelve

Living Large Again

I never got to goal weight. During my final stay at the Rice House, my mother got colon cancer, and I was devastated. My father was always the ill one in our family; my mother was never sick. I thought of her as invincible. I was torn between going home and being with my mother and staying at the Rice House to get to goal weight—between what I desperately wanted to accomplish and what my family needed of me. It is the core tension of the women at the Rice House: their individual needs versus the needs of their families back home. Dr. Kempner, of course, urged me to stay and get to goal weight. He told me that if I only stuck it out and lost the rest of my weight, my whole family and I would benefit. A nurse at the Rice House told me that I could always come back to the Rice House and finish what I started, that I should go home and be with my mother.

I chose to go to my mother, and for a summer I stayed with her in Rochester, Minnesota, while she was a patient at the Mayo Clinic. She was on chemotherapy for a year, and her treatments were successful. While I was in Rochester, I didn't have a car, so I would be forced to walk as exercise. I walked everywhere: to the Clinic, to the grocery store, and to the drugstore for medications for my mother. I bought a pedometer and logged my miles each day, which averaged eight. I ate at the cafeteria at one of the hospitals that provided low-fat, low-sodium meals. Of course, they were not as low-calorie or low-sodium as Rice House meals, but they were the best I could do in Rochester.

An incident occurred that brought all of my feelings about eating into stark light. My dad was visiting from Missouri, and he and my mother got into an argument about money. There was nothing unusual about that; they fought often and always over the same things. I was used to their fighting. It was the background music of my childhood. For some reason, this time I just couldn't take it, and I placed myself between my mother—standing there with her gaping wound from her recent cancer surgery—and my angry father.

I made my father leave. My mother was extremely upset with me and my father, but instead of talking about it, she wanted to go out and eat. We went to a Chinese restaurant, but neither one of us felt like eating. For the first time in my life, I couldn't eat away what I was feeling. My mother, as a result of her treatment, was too nauseated to even look at the food. Still, she refused to give up and, after the uneaten meal was carried away, we stopped by a candy shop and she bought the old familiar white bag of chocolates. I knew what kind they were without looking: thick dark chocolate, waxy on the outside with creamy, sweet white centers. When any anger looms in our family, we go out to dinner, eat in large amounts, and finish it off with that universal soother—chocolate. That behavior didn't seem to bother anyone but me. I was the fat one, the one who carried all the weight.

I remembered when, as a little girl in Kansas City, I sat in the car eating cream puffs with my upset mother. I can still recollect the look, smell, and taste of those cream puffs, and how the first couple of bites would catch in my throat and form a knot. I would panic and feel that the cream puff was going to suffocate me. But then I would relax and the creamy part would melt down my throat. I would gulp the crisp, flaky crust the rest of the way down. My hands, face, clothes, and even my shoes would have smudges of powered sugar on them.

Where was my dad during these escapes to the bakery? He must have stayed home. Where was my sister? Perhaps she had escaped out the door on one of her extended walks, or maybe she had climbed a tree. I have vivid memories of my father making my sister get down from trees. Me, I was in the car, in a private ceremony, eating because the food was lovely and secret and would obliterate any tension at home. By the time we got home, everything was calm. No words were spoken. Nobody wanted to stir things up. I just got fatter.

Years later, when I was an adult living in my own apartment in another town, my mother would often call and suggest that we get together. We would spend the day shopping, and it always ended with a chocolate rush. This time, the little white bags were from the Fannie Mae candy outlet center. There was a store not too far from my parents' home, and it had a big sign that read Rejects Available Here—candy that didn't make the cut to go into a Fannie Mae gift box. When my mother saw that sign, she would pull into the parking lot and buy a couple of bags of rejects. These candies had dark chocolate on the outside and a creamy white center, but because they were rejects, the creamy part bulged out in places. The candies looked like someone had squashed them. It didn't matter. We ate them anyway. After my the third or fourth candy, my head would begin to ache from the sugar, but I continued to eat. By this time, my father had grown to love candy too, and he would eagerly look forward to the white paper bag my mom always brought him. I never said a word on these candy binges. I sat on the passenger's side of the car and ate one bonbon after another. The only sound was the rustling of candy wrappers.

At the end of the summer, I left my mother in Rochester and went back to Durham. Despite my best intentions, when I got on the scales at the Rice House, my weight was up fourteen pounds.

I entered graduate school that fall and worked part time. My weight went up and down, around twenty-eight pounds every four months or so. Sometimes I would eat three meals a day. Sometimes I wouldn't eat for days, and then when I did return to eating, I would only eat the food that I really craved and only enough to make my stomach stop growling. I would eat a couple of bites and toss the rest of the food away. I had three sets of clothes in the closet, for my low, middle, and high weights. I rejoined Weight

Watchers and went back to Overeaters Anonymous, but it wasn't until I went back on program at the Rice House that I lost thirty pounds and maintained the loss.

I kept my hundred pounds off for a decade, and sometimes I lost even more weight. A year or two after graduate school I lost an additional thirty pounds, but it was very hard to maintain and I hovered around a total one-hundred to 120-pound loss.

Keeping the weight off was a full-time job. I worked part time to support my full-time weight maintenance. On the average, I exercised four hours a day—two hours of aerobics and two hours of continuous walking—and ate a maximum of twelve hundred calories a day. I did not eat meat, cheese, or canned or frozen foods. My only indulgence was two cups of coffee with a half a teaspoon of sugar and a tablespoon of half-and-half. I measured and weighed everything I ate and drank. I would exercise so hard that I got chills and felt sick after a session. I was always hungry, and my stomach ached. I ate Tums and Tagamet to quell the continuous churning and incessant heartburn.

I met a lot of nice people and dated many of them, but didn't want to get too involved with anyone. My idea of a perfect relationship was one that started on a Thursday night and ended on the following Sunday morning. I loathed commitment because commitment meant that I would have to consider someone else's feelings and needs before my own, and if I did that, I knew that the weight would zoom right back on. No nondieter would understand the fanatic devotion I had to keeping my weight off. Ricers told me not to get married because I wouldn't have a chance in hell of keeping it off, let alone losing any more weight. Dr. Kempner used to lament that his fat female patients would get thin, get married, have children, and get fat again. I was determined that I was going to escape that fate.

Yet I knew that being married to weight maintenance was a limited and lonely life. To confront my fear of commitment, I started therapy, and little by little I allowed some relationships to develop. But if things got really serious, I would withdraw or begin having panic attacks. Once my doctor prescribed medication so I could continue going out with a man I had been dating. He even stayed longer than a weekend, and I survived. With a lot of time and effort, my fears began to subside. I gained a little weight, but went right back to the Rice House and took it off. I got a full-time job, and my cut down my exercise to two hours: one hour of aerobics and one hour of walking.

In 1995, I met my husband on a blind date arranged by a co-worker of mine. She described me to my future husband as someone who "was really overweight, but had a pretty face." It was the same description I had had when I was a hundred and thirty pounds heavier. In fact, it was the same description I had had all of my life. Again, I was reminded of my interview with Susan Tucker where she said that "one is not considered thin unless one gets below 140 pounds." To the world, I was still fat.

Two weeks after we met, David proposed to me. My immediate reaction was that he was some kind of nut and I should get an unlisted phone number, but he persisted, and I let go of my fears and fell in love. David had been married before and was familiar with the devastating effects of obesity. He revealed to me that at the time of her death, his wife had weighed 315 pounds. He said he was never physically repulsed by her appearance, and I figured if he could deal with that amount of weight, then he could deal with mine.

I convinced myself that I would keep off the weight. I told myself that I would prepare healthy, low-fat meals that David and his two skinny boys would enjoy. As a family, we would exercise together, perhaps play tennis, or golf, or bike around a lake somewhere. We would hike in the woods, surf at the coast, and ski in mountains. I even returned to the Rice House a month before the wedding so I could knock off another twenty pounds.

After I was married, I quit my job and moved with David to Winston-Salem, about an hour and a half's drive from Durham. I thought that if things got tough and my weight started to come back, I could drive back to Durham for a couple of days. How hard could that be? But I knew I wouldn't need to go back to the Rice House, because I was going to eat healthy and make sure everyone else did too.

Within a week of my marriage, I was preparing fried chicken

and biscuits, cookies, cakes, and pies, as well as buying gallons of soda and bushels of potato chips. I would go to three different grocery stores in one day just to get all of the supplies we needed. Weekends were spent at food warehouses like Sam's Club, where I would pile up a cart with cases of Coke, giant bags of chips, pounds of frozen meat, and gallons of whole milk, butter, and ice cream. I, who for a decade hadn't entered a kitchen, cooked a meal, or shopped at a grocery store, was now expected to make breakfasts and dinners and snacks. It was frightening how much food one grown man and two growing boys could eat. They would eat a meal and an hour later eat another one. They always had something to eat in their hands and food in their mouths. Our family room was littered with empty soda bottles, crumpled potato chip bags, McDonald's styrofoam boxes, and empty pizza containers. I was surrounded by all the wrong foods and by people who ate with abandon.

I learned that my parents' approach to eating was not as dysfunctional as I had thought. David also ate for comfort, and to alleviate boredom, frustration, and just for the hell of it. He simply didn't get fat from it. He couldn't understand why I had to be so vigilant about what I ate. He thought that a moderate approach would keep the weight off.

We attended social eating situations where he ate what he wanted, and I drank ice water. Everywhere, I saw people consume gobs of high-fat foods and wash it all down with what seemed like vats of beer. I was expected to cook but not partake, attend but not eat. It was maddening. I called up old Ricer friends and they basically said "I told you so." They couldn't keep the weight off once they got home, so why did I think that I could? But I did think I could do it. I was convinced that I could be one of the few who kept it off.

Despite all my good intentions, the weight crept back up. I gained eleven pounds the first month of my marriage. I resented my new family for being able to eat anything they liked at all hours of the day and night, while I was supposed to be satisfied with a bowl of rice and two fruits. I had to cut my exercise back because I just didn't have the time or energy to devote to it. There were football and soccer practices to attend, Boy Scout bake drives, school assemblies, church dinners, parties, company picnics, birthday celebrations, holidays, Sunday dinners, and other eating events in which I was required to participate. I felt like I had been hit by a blast furnace. The only thing I knew to do was to go back to Durham.

I went back to the Rice House four months after I was married. I had gained twenty-five pounds. It took me a month to lose that weight and about a week to regain it once I returned home. I just could not keep it off.

I joined Weight Watchers and Physicians Weight Loss Center, took diet medications and antidepressants, and joined the YMCA. I even went to a Chinese acupuncturist who said I had an imbalance and prescribed bitter Chinese herbs, which I dutifully gulped each morning. Nothing worked. The weight just kept on coming.

When my mother called, she would always tell me not to "eat anything good." My sister told me, "Don't do it. Don't eat anything." I was in a panic. And all the time my family couldn't figure out why I just couldn't lose weight. David had a fat wife again, when he'd married a merely overweight one.

I learned that I am no different from any other dieters. I thought I was because I thought I had incorporated the principles of dieting into my very soul. I knew what to eat, when to eat, and how to eat. I meditated, exercised, and journaled, and the weight kept coming.

My total weight gain since my marriage is forty pounds. I diet and exercise, and if I'm lucky, I maintain. Sometimes I lose a few pounds and sometimes I gain. Once I was hospitalized with a bad stomach virus and lost eighteen pounds. I gained it back in week.

I have learned a lot of things on my dieting journey. I learned that, when it comes to weight, the world really is as superficial and shallow as I assumed. I also learned that weight is a relative concept to some people. What would be considered fat to others seems merely overweight to David and even svelte to fellow Ricers. David would prefer a thin wife, and the children would like a thin mother, but they got a fat one, and they can learn to live with that. However, thin is just better, no matter how much I try to challenge that stereotype. The world really does love you thin and hate you fat.

I miss Durham. I miss the acceptance and love I felt from Ricers. I miss the sexual freedom, the body freedom I had with them. I miss all that desire: the desire for more, the abundant flesh, the feeling that I am wonderful as is—not twenty pounds less from now, but wonderful in the very moment. And the unspoken understanding of what it is like to be caught between two desires—one to be thin and healthy and acceptable to the dominant culture, and one to eat without boundaries, eat without always calculating the fat, sodium, and calorie content of every morsel. I have always had this conflict between reality and desire. The reality is I can't eat what I want. I must always have less than I desire.

I remember an incident from when I was about ten years old. My mother and I were sitting in a restaurant. I looked at the menu and declared that I wanted a cheeseburger, onion rings, and a Coke. My mother scolded me and said that I shouldn't have what I wanted. I should eat what the cute little girl at a nearby table was eating. I turned my head to see a child about my age—petite, with her hair slicked up into a brown bun on the top of her pointy head. Her spindly little legs were crossed at her ankles. She wore a girly type of dress with smocking across the bodice and puffy sleeves. Even her white ankle socks had ruffles on them. The kid was eating a small salad.

I remember thinking that she looked downtrodden, timid, and hungry. Her mother sat across from her and was talking and waving her hands in the air. Maybe she was telling the kid not to eat so much of the salad. I turned my attention back to my mother. Her round face was full of concern. I looked down at my bulky body—my rumpled pedal-pushers that wouldn't stay down and my socks that wouldn't stay up. My wild hair escaping the confines of my ponytail. When our waiter reappeared, I, with authority, ordered the cheeseburger. My mother shook her head.

I am grown up now and know the consequences of eating what I desire. To eat with pleasure is something I will never experience again except in stolen moments, and even then it is with the guilt and knowledge that I will pay for each swallow, pay at the scale. So

I eat the miniature Snickers bar and pair it with a Diet Coke, hoping for some kind of balance between desire and discipline.

Yet food seems to have lost its wonderful pull. This sounds like a positive thing, but it is not. Food to me was always the secret lover, the one thing that could soothe me, love me, and transport me to another place. An alcoholic that I met while on program told me that she drank until she felt balanced. At that point, whatever was bothering her fell away, and the world became brighter. That was the way I felt about food. It was a pleasurable painkiller that I could buy anywhere at any time. Now it doesn't do that for me, doesn't work like a drug. It's just food. When I an angry, upset, happy, nervous, or just want to float away, food no longer makes me feel better. Sometimes I feel abandoned by food.

But a miraculous thing has happened. I've made a truce with myself about who I am and the defining role fat has played in my life. I credit going through the torture of the Rice Diet as forcing this change in me. I am a changed person because of the Rice Diet, because of the program itself, because of the weight loss, and because of the stories and experiences of other Dieters. I am a better person, too, because I have proved to myself and to those who know me that I can do a very difficult thing. I can challenge myself, and I can succeed. Since I have completed my tour of duty at the Rice House, I believe I have the strength to do anything. Yes, I have regained forty pounds, but I have kept off sixty, and the really wonderful thing is I don't think of myself as fat. I don't think of weight at all. I just live my life.

Sometimes when I overhear a fat remark somewhere I will react, but not usually. When I am at exercise class some chubby will comment on a thin passerby and nudge me and wish out loud that we could be like that person. I am amused at this. Strangers have no idea what I have done to lose weight. When a doctor admonishes me about being fat I look at him and smile.

The most amazing thing about my whole dieting experience is not my weight loss, but how I feel about myself. I have left my fat identity behind. Clearly I am fat, just not as fat as I once was—but I don't view myself as such. And I like my body. It brings pleasure to me and gives it to others. Oddly, and refreshingly, I don't define myself by weight. I wasted most of my life being absolutely dominated by weight and its repercussions. My dieting experience brought forth a revolution of self. I have moved on from my old identity of a fat lady waiting to be granted validity through weight loss to a new identity of transcendence. I now view myself as a person—strong, capable, and worthy.

notes

1. Kenneth Meyer [pseud.]. Tape-recorded interview. Durham, N.C., 18 Jan 1992.

2. Meyer, interview.

3. Karen Reeves [pseud.]. Tape-recorded interview. Durham, N.C., 24 May 1992.

4. Judy Moscovitz. Tape-recorded interview. Durham, N.C., 17 Feb 1992.

5. Robert J. Kuczmarski, Dr. PhD, RD; Katherine M. Flegal, PhD; Stephen M. Campbell, MSH; Clifford L. Johnson, MSPH. *Journal of the American Medical Association* 272, no. 3 (20 Jul 1994): 205–239.

6. Roberta Pollack Seid. *Never Too Thin: Why Women Are at War With Their Bodies* (New York: Prentice Hall Press, 1989): 33.

7. Walter J. Kempner, MD. *Bulletin of the Walter Kempner Foundation* 272, no. 3 (Dec 1962).

8. Ethylene Cole. As told to Jean Renfro, Durham, N.C., 15 Aug 1988.

9. Jim Wise. "Kempner Made Durham, Rice Diet Synonymous," *The Herald Sun*. 12 Oct 1999: 12–14.

10. Eugene A. Stead, MD. "A prospective," *Archives of Internal Medicine* 133 (May 1974).

11. James F. Gifford. "Rice and Health at Duke," *Duke Dialogue* (16 Nov 1990): 9.

12. Rodger Lyle Brown. "Fat City," *Atlanta Constitution*. 15 Mar 1992: M1–M6.

13. Debbie Moose. "A Losing Proposition," *News and Observer*. 2 Mar 1992b: 7C.

14. Kae Enright, MD. Tape-recorded interview. Durham, N.C., 20 Sep 1990.

15. The complaint filed November 4, 1993 in Durham County in the General Court of Justice Superior Court Division 93 CVS 04014. Sharon Ryan (Plaintiff) v. Walter Kempner, MD, The Rice Diet, Inc., d/b/a/ Kempner Clinic, Duke University, Duke University Medical Center, and Medical Private Diagnostic Clinic (Defendants), page 5, article 18: "For the next eighteen years, until mid-1987, plaintiff functioned as Kempner's virtual sex slave/servant."

16. The *Durham Herald-Sun* and the Raleigh *News and Observer* widely reported the details of this lawsuit in 1993 and 1994. For a retrospective see, "Suit reveals Kempner's guarded private life. Rice Diet doctor was brilliant, generous, strange." Chris O'Brien and Wendy Hower, staff writers. *News and Observer,* Raleigh, N.C. 19 October 1997.

17. Al Goldstein. "Sex in Fat City. A True Story of Beauty and the Obese," *Penthouse Magazine,* 1984

18. Robert Rosati, MD. "Rap at the Rice House" Event. Durham, N.C., 20 Feb 1992.

19. Judy Moscovitz. *The Rice Diet Report* (New York: G.P. Putnam's and Sons, 1986).

20. Burr Snider. "Fat City," *Esquire Magazine.* Mar 1973: 112–182.

21. Ibid.

22. Ibid.

bibliography

Adams, Alicia [pseud.]. Interview by author. Tape recording. Durham, N.C., 1 October 1995.

Adams, Timothy [pseud.]. Interview by author. Tape recording. Durham, N.C., 5 February 1992.

Alcoholics Anonymous. *The Big Book: The Basic Text for Alcoholic Anonymous*. New York: AA World Services, 1976.

Alexander, Mark [pseud.]. Interview by author. Tape recording. Durham, N.C., 4 July 1995.

Alexander, Roy. *The Ricers' Guide to Work and Play in Durham*. Durham, N.C. Duke University Medical Center, 1980.

Anderson, Sharon [pseud.]. Interview by author. Tape recording. Durham, N.C., 15 January 2000.

Apte, Mahadev L. *Humor and Laughter: An Anthropological Approach*. Ithaca: Cornell University Press, 1985.

A Season in Hell. Hohokus, N.J.: New Day Films. Aired on PBS's *P.O.V.* 20 July 1992.

Bararres, Kelly [pseud.]. Interview by author. Tape recording. Durham, N.C., 5 August 1997.

Baucman, Eddie [pseud.]. Interview by author. Tape recording. Durham, N.C., 12 April 1992.

Bauman, Charlotte, Paula Hyman, and Sonya Michel. "Pearls Around the Neck, A Stone upon the Heart: Becoming an American Lady." In: *Immigrant Women*, edited by Maxine Schwarts Seller. Philadelphia: Temple University Press, 1981, 140–149.

Bauman, Richard. "Differential Identity and the Social Base of Folklore," *Journal of American Folklore* 84 (1971): 41–42.

Ben-Amos, Dan. "Toward a Definition of Folklore in Context," *Journal of American Folklore* 84 (1971): 3–15.

Bennet, Leslie [pseud.]. Interview by author. Tape recording. Durham, N.C., 6 May 1992.

Bennet, William. *The Dieter's Dilemma: Eating Less and Weighing More.* New York: Basic Books, 1982.

Bennion, Lynn J., Edwin L. Bierman, and James M. Ferguson. *Straight Talk About Weight Control: Taking Off Pounds and Keeping Them Off.* Mount Vernon, N.Y.: Consumers' Union, 1991.

Beru, Rhonda [pseud.]. Interview by author. Tape recording. Durham, N.C., 16 June 1999.

Black, Evan Imber, and Janine Roberts. *Rituals for Our Times.* New York: HarperCollins, 1992.

Blackwell, Karen [pseud.]. Interview by author. Tape recording. Durham, N.C., 1 November 1998.

Blum, David [pseud.]. Interview by author. Tape recording. Durham, N.C., 10 July 1992.

Bly, Robert. *Iron John: A Book About Men.* Reading, Mass.: Addison-Wesley Publishing, 1990.

Body Dismorphic Disorder. Transcript. Livingston: Burrelle's Information Services. Aired on CBS's *48 Hours.* 3 June 1992.

Boorstin, Daniel J. *The Creators: A History of Heroes of the Imagination.* New York: Random House, 1992.

Boyd, Lee [pseud.]. Interview by author. Tape recording. Durham, N.C., 27 January 1992.

Brooks, Tom [pseud.]. Interview by author. Tape recording. Durham, N.C., 20 March 1992.

Brown, Rodger Lyle. "Fat City," *Atlanta Constitution.* 15 March 1992: M1–M6.

Brownmiller, Susan. *Femininity.* New York: Simon & Schuster, 1984.

Brumberg, Joan Jacobs. *Fasting Girls: The Emergence of Anorexia Nervosa as a Modern Disease.* Cambridge: Harvard University Press, 1998.

Calanero, Joyce [pseud.]. Interview by author. Tape recording. Durham, N.C., 14 August 1995.

Callaway, Wayne C., and Dan Kirschenbaum. "Should Obesity Often Be Treated as an Eating Disorder?" *Washington Post.* 21 January 1992: 13.

Camp, Charles. *American Foodways: What, When, Why, and How We Eat in America.* Little Rock: August House, 1989.

Campbell, Joseph. *Myths to Live By*. New York: Bantam Books, 1972.

Campbell, Joseph. *The Hero with a Thousand Faces*. Princeton: Princeton University Press, 1973.

Canter, Kym. "Full Strength Fashion," *Washington Post Magazine*. September 1992: 11–21.

Catesano, Linda, and Larry Catesano [pseuds.]. Interview by author. Tape recording. Durham, N.C., 19 May 1992.

Center for Living Information Packet. Durham, N.C.: Duke University Medical Center, 1992.

Chapkis, Wendy. *Beauty Secret: Women and the Politics of Appearance*. Boston: South End, 1986.

Chiesa, Elizabeth [pseud.]. Interview by author. Tape recording. Durham, N.C., 1 July 1995.

Chernin, Kim. *The Hungry Self: Women, Eating, and Identity*. New York: Random House, 1985.

Clements, William M. "Public Testimony as Oral Performance," *Linguistica Biblica* 47, 1980: 21–32.

Clements, William M. "Conversions and Communitas." *Western Folklore*, 35 1976: 35–45.

Clements, William M. "Personal Narrative: The Interview, Context and Quest of Tradition," *Western Folklore* 39, 1980: 106–112.

Cole, Ethylene. As told to Jean Renfro, Durham, N.C., 15 Aug 1988

Cole, Thomas R. *The Journey of Life: A Cultural History of Aging in America*. Cambridge: Cambridge University Press, 1992.

Collins, Linda, and Rita Collins [pseuds.]. Interview by author. Tape recording. Durham, N.C., 13 September 1990.

Conners, Stephen [pseud.]. Interview by author. Tape recording. Durham, N.C., 23 September 1995.

Cox, Harvey. *The Feast of Fools: A Theological Essay on Festivity and Fantasy*. Cambridge: Harvard University Press, 1969.

Craft, Christine. *Too Old, Too Ugly and Not Deferential to Men*. New York: Dell Books, 1988.

Crowder, Pat [pseud.]. Interview by author. Tape recording. Durham, N.C., 8 March 1992.

Daly, Carol [pseud.]. Tape-recorded interview, Durham, N.C., 6 October 1990.

David, Angela. *Women, Culture and Politics*. New York: Random House, 1989.

Dellon, Alexa [pseud.]. Interview by author. Tape recording. Durham, N.C., 14 April 2000.

DeNatale, Douglas. "The Dissembling Line: Industrial Pranks in a

North Carolina Textile Mill." In: *Arts in Earnest*, edited by Daniel W. Patterson and Charles G. Zug III, Durham, N.C.: Duke University Press, 1990, 251–276.

Demetrakopoulos, Stephanie. *Listening to Our Bodies: The Rebirth of Feminine Wisdom*. Boston: Beacon, 1983.

Ditmar, Mary [pseud.]. Interview by author. Tape recording. Durham, N.C., 24 September 1990.

Dixon, Sloane [pseud.]. Interview by author. Tape recording. Durham, N.C., 12 August 1995.

Doheny, Kathleen. The New Diet Drugs. *Allure*. October 1992: 80–85.

Douglas, Mary W. *Natural Symbols, Explorations in Cosmology*. New York: Pantheon Books, 1982.

Druck, Kena, and James C. Simmons. *The Secrets Men Keep: Breaking the Silence Barrier.* Garden City, N.J.: Doubleday, 1985.

Dworkin, Andrea. *Pornography: Men Possessing Women*. New York: Putnam, 1981.

Emerson, Gloria. *Some American Men*. New York: Simon & Schuster, 1985.

Enright, Kae, MD. Interview by author. Tape recording. Durham, N.C., 20 September 1990.

Estes, Clarissa Pinkola. *Women Who Run with the Wolves: Myths and Stories of the Wild Woman Archetype*. New York: Ballantine Books, 1992.

Faludi, Susan. *Backlash: The Undeclared War Against American Women*. New York: Crown Publishers, 1991.

Felcher, Abby [pseud.]. Interview by author. Tape recording. Durham, N.C., 18 September 1993.

Fishbine, Joel. [pseud.] Interview by author. Tape recording. Durham, N.C., 14 February 1993.

Firestone, Shulasmith. *The Dialectic of Sex*. New York: Bantam Books, 1971.

Fisher, Walter R. "Narration as a Human Communication Paradigm," *Communication Monographs* 51 (1984): 1–19.

Fox-Genevese, Elizabeth. *Feminism Without Illusions: A Critique of Individualism*. Chapel Hill: University of North Carolina Press, 1991.

Franklin, John. *Writing for Story: Craft Secrets of Dramatic Nonfiction by a Two-Time Pulitzer Prize Winner.* New York: Penguin Books, 1986.

Fredrick, John [pseud.]. Interview by author. Tape recording. Durham, N.C., 24 November 1995.

Freedman, Rita. *Beauty Bound: Why We Pursue the Myth in the Mirror.* Lexington, Ky.: D.C. Heath, 1986.

Friedan, Betty. *The Feminine Mystique*. London: Penguin Books, 1992.

French, Marilyn. *The War Against Women.* New York: Summit Books, 1992.

Friends in Recovery. *The Twelve Steps—A Spiritual Journey.* San Diego: Recovery Publications, 1988.

Furst, Lilian R., and Peter W. Graham, eds. *Disorderly Eaters: Texts in Self-Empowerment.* University Park: Pennsylvania State University Press, 1992.

Geertz, Clifford. *The Interpretation of Cultures: Selected Essays.* New York: Basic Books, 1973.

Georges, Robert A. Toward an Understanding of Storytelling Events. *Journal of American Folklore* 82 (1969): 313–328.

Gifford, James F. "Rice and Health at Duke," *Duke Dialogue* 16 (November 1990): 9.

Gilday, Katherine. *Famine Within.* Kandor Productions and Telefilm of Canada (1992), 120 min.

Gilligan, Carol. *In a Different Voice: Psychological Theory and Women's Development.* Cambridge: Harvard University Press, 1982.

Ginsberg, Faye. "When the Subject is Women: Encounters with Syrian Jewish Women," *Journal of American Folklore* 100 (1987): 540–547.

Goldman, Sylvia [pseud.]. Tape-recorded interview, Chapel Hill, N.C., 21 May 1990.

Goldstein, Al. "Sex in Fat City: A True Story of Beauty and the Obese," *Penthouse.* November (1984): 114–118.

Gordon, Suzanne. *Prisoners of Men's Dreams: Striking Out for a New Feminine Future.* Boston: Little, Brown, 1991.

Gough, Peter [pseud.]. Interview by author. Tape recording. Durham, N.C., 22 March 1992.

Grant, Elizabeth [pseud.]. Interview by author. Tape recording. Durham, N.C., 25 March 1992.

Gras, Stevie. "Secret of Her Success: Personal triumphs of Weight-Loss Winners." *Weight Watchers Magazine.* January (1993): 62–65.

Green, Ann [pseud.]. Interview by author. Tape recording. Durham, N.C., 24 January 1992.

Greer, Germaine. *The Madwoman's Underclothes.* New York: Atlantic Monthly Press, 1986.

Greer, Germaine. *The Female Eunuch.* London: Paladin Grafton Books, 1985.

Greeson, Janet. *It's Not What You're Eating, It's What's Eating You.* New York: Simon & Schuster, 1990.

Griffith, John [pseud.]. Interview by author. Tape recording. Durham, N.C., 14 December 1990.

Grossman, Sylvia [pseud.]. Interview by author. Tape recording. Durham, N.C., 6 October 1990.

Groves, Irene [pseud.]. Interview by author. Tape recording. Durham, N.C., 2 August 1990.

Gruber, Brent [pseud.]. Interview by author. Tape recording. Durham, N.C., 4 March 1993.

Gruian, Michael. *The Prince and the King*. Los Angeles: Jeremy P. Tarcher, 1992.

Hamilton, Michael, MD. Written interview. Durham, N.C., 26 March 1992.

Heer, Friedrich. *The Medieval World.* Translated by Janet Sonheimer. New York: New American Library, 1962.

Heiman, Heather. "Distorted Images." *Currents*. November 1992: 7–9.

Heiman, Kae [pseud.]. Interview by author. Tape recording. Chapel Hill, N.C., 3 March 1992.

Heimel, Cynthia. "My Life as a Tank." *Playboy.* December 1992: 40.

Henderson, Gene. "How to Become a Christian." In *Pathways of Faith: Adult Bible Teacher.* Nashville: Sunday School Board of the Southern Baptist Convention, 1993.

Hirshfield, Barbara [pseud.]. Interview by author. Tape recording. Durham, N.C., 7 July 1992.

Hirschman, Jane R. *Overcoming Overeating: Living Free in a World of Food.* New York: Ballantine Books, 1989.

Hobgood, Bob [pseud.]. Interview by author. Tape recording. Durham, N.C., 1 October 1993.

Hollandsworth, Skip. "Hard Bodies, Soft Touch," *Self.* May 1992: 90–91.

Holleman, Jack [pseud.]. Interview by author. Tape recording. Durham, N.C., 6 October 1992.

Horace, Henry [pseud.]. Interview by author. Tape recording. Winston-Salem, N.C., 8 March 1996.

Houston, Pam. "The Biggest Sin," *Allure*. December 1992: 110–11.

Jacobs, Sarah [pseud.]. Interview by author. Tape recording. Durham, N.C., 3 May 1992.

Jenkins, Annie [pseud.]. Interview by author. Tape recording. Durham, N.C., 3 May 1992.

Johnson, Joe [pseud.]. Interview by author. Tape recording. Durham, N.C., 3 May 1992.

Joyner, Charles W. "A Model for the Analysis of Folklore Performance in Historical Context," *Journal of American Folklore* 88 (1975): 254–265.

Kalan, Jane Rachel. *The Special Relationship Between Women and Food.* Englewood Cliffs, N.J.: Prentice-Hall, 1980.

Kaskew, Paul, and Cynthia H. Adams. *When Food Is a Four-Letter Word.* Englewood Cliffs, N.J.: Prentice Hall, 1984.

Kaufman, P. "Health," *Vogue.* March 1992: 243.

Kellor, Sam [pseud.]. Interview by author. Tape recording. Durham, N.C., 23 March 1992.

Kellor, Sam [pseud.]. Interview by author. Tape recording. Durham, N.C., 1 March 1992.

Kempner, Walter J., MD. "Treatment of Heart and Kidney Disease with the Rice Diet," *Annals of Internal Medicine* (31 November 1949): 821–856.

Kempner, Walter J., MD. "Obesity," *Bulletin of the Walter J. Kempner Foundation.* 3 December 1962: 17–20.

Kempner, Walter J., MD. *Bulletin of the Walter Kempner Foundation* 272, no. 3. Dec 1962.

Kerby, Anthony P. *Narrative and the Self.* Bloomington: Indiana University Press, 1991.

Knott, Doris [pseud.]. Interview by author. Tape recording. Durham, N.C., 11 September 1994.

Kolata, Gina. "Ridiculed and Scorned: Overweight People Face Abuse, Discrimination," *Durham Herald-Sun.* 28 November 1992: G1–G2.

Kopecky, Gini. "The Season of Doubt: Girls May Lose Self-Confidence in Adolescence," *Kansas City Star.* 16 December 1992: F1–F4.

Kota, Dennis [pseud.]. Interview by author. Tape recording. Durham, N.C., 7 March 1989.

Krool-Smith, Stephen Jay. "The Testimony as Performance," *Journal for the Scientific Study of Religion* 19 (1980):16–25.

Kuczmarski, Robert J. Dr. PhD; Katherine M. Flegal, PhD; Stephen M. Campbell, MSH; Clifford L. Johnson, MSPH. "Increasing Prevalence of Overweight among U.S. Adults: The National Health and Nutrition Examination Surveys 1960–1991," *Journal of the American Medical Association* 272 no. 3 (20 July 1994): 205–239.

Labov, William. *Language in the Inner City.* Philadelphia: University of Pennsylvania Press.

Lang, Susan S. "Are You Ready to Lose Weight?" *New Woman.* June 1992: 119–121.

Langellier, Kristin M. "Personal Narratives: Perspectives on Theory and Research," *Text and Performance Quarterly* 9 (1989): 243–276.

Lasch, Christopher. *The Culture of Narcissism: American Life in the Age of Diminishing Expectations.* New York: W. W. Norton, 1979.

Leland, John, and Elizabeth Nenard. "Back to Twiggy," *Newsweek*. 1 February 1993: 64–65.

Lenz, Elinor, and Barbara Myerhoff. *The Feminization of America: How Women's Values Are Changing Our Public and Private Lives*. Los Angeles: Jeremy P. Tarcher, 1985.

Linde, Charlotte. *Life Stories: The Creation of Coherence*. New York: Oxford University Press, 1993.

Littleton, Susan [pseud.]. Conversation with author, Durham, N.C., 3 November 1995.

Livingston, Ellen [pseud.]. Interview by author. Tape recording. Durham, N.C., 28 August 1998.

Long, Patricia. "The Great Weight Debate." *Health*. March 1992: 42–47.

Lewinsohn, Richard. *A History of Sexual Customs*. Translated by Alexander Mayce. New York: Harper & Brothers, 1958.

Marletti, Linda [pseud.]. Interview by author. Tape recording. Durham, N.C., 15 January 1990.

Mayfield, Ellen [pseud.]. Interview by author. Tape recording. Chapel Hill, N.C., 2 April 1992.

McCarl, Robert Jr. "Smokejumper Initiation—Ritualized Communication in a Modern Occupation," *Journal of American Folklore* 94 (1981): 58–85.

McCarl, Robert Jr. "Occupational Folklore: A Theoretical Hypothesis," In: *Working American: Contemporary Approaches to Occupational Folklife,* edited by Robert Byington. Los Angeles: California Folklore Society, 1978.

McCarthy, Dorothy [pseud.]. Interview by author. Tape recording. Durham, N.C., 18 December 1995.

McFarland, Barbara. *Shame and Body Image: Culture and the Compulsive Overeater.* Deerfield Beach: Deerfield, 1990.

McKlellan, Diana. "In Your Face," *Washingtonian Magazine*. October 1992: 80–88.

Melamed, Elissa. *Mirror, Mirror: The Terror of Not Being Young*. New York: Linden Press and Simon & Schuster, 1983.

Meyer, Kenneth [pseud.]. Interview by author. Tape recording. Durham, N.C., 18 January 1992.

Miles, Rosalind. *Love, Sex, Death, and the Making of the Male*. New York: Summit Books, 1991.

Millman, Marcia. *Such a Pretty Face: Being Fat in America*. New York: W.W. Norton, 1980.

Moe, Susan Spence. "Dieting with Rice," *Raleigh News & Observer.* 6 March 1977: E1, E7.

Moffitt, Sylvia [pseud.]. Interview by author. Tape recording. Durham, N.C., 30 May 1992.

Moose, Debbie. "A Losing Proposition," *News and Observer.* 2 Mar 1992b: 7C.

Moose, Debbie. "Fat City," *News & Observer.* 1 Mar 1992a:1, E6.

Moose, Debbie. "Living Off the Fat of the Land," *Raleigh News & Observer.* 3 March 1992b: E1–E6.

Morgan, Robin. *The Anatomy of Freedom: Feminism, Physics, and Global Politics.* Garden City, N.J.: Anchor, 1982.

Moscovitz, Judy. *The Rice Diet Report.* New York: G. P. Putman's Sons, 1986.

Moscovitz, Judy. *The Dieter's Companion.* New York: Avon Books, 1989.

Moscovitz, Judy. Interview by author. Tape recording. Durham, N.C., 17 February 1992.

Mullen, Patrick. *Listening to Old Voices: Folklore, Life Stories, and the Elderly.* Urbana: University of Illinois Press, 1992.

Musanti, Gerard [pseud.]. Written interview by author. Durham, N.C., 7 March 1992.

Myherhoff, Barbara. *Number Our Days.* New York: Simon & Schuster, 1979.

Myherhoff, Barbara. "Rites of Passage: Process and Paradox." In: *Celebration: Studies in Restivity and Ritual,* edited by Victor Turner. Washington, D.C.: Smithsonian Institution Press, 1982: 109–139.

Neal, Norman [pseud.]. Interview by author. Tape recording. Durham, N.C., 5 January 1992.

Noorman, Licke. "Coedsel als Minnaar-Durham: Domein voor dikkerds," *NRC Handelsbkad.* 10 October 1992: 5.

O'Brien, Chris, and Wendy Hower. "Suit reveals Kempner's guarded private life: Rice Diet doctor was brilliant, generous, strange," *Raleigh News & Observer.* 19 October 1997: A1, A10.

Orbach, Suzie. *Fat Is a Feminist Issue: A Self-Help Guide for the Compulsive Overeater.* New York: Berkeley Publishing Corporation, 1979.

Oring, Elliot. "Jokes and the Discourse on Disaster," *Journal of American Folklore* 100 (1987): 277–286.

Overeaters Anonymous. *The Twelve Steps of Overeaters Anonymous.* Torrance, Calif.: Overeaters Anonymous Press, 1990.

Overeaters Anonymous. *Overeaters Anonymous.* Torrance, Calif.: Overeaters Anonymous Press, 1980.

Owens, Cynthia [pseud.]. Interview by author. Tape recording. Durham, N.C., 2 February 2000.

Paglia, Camille. *Sexual Personae: Art and Decadence from Nefertiti to Emily Dickinson*. New York: Random House, 1990.

Patel, Nathan [pseud.]. Interview by author. Tape recording. Durham, N.C., 30 July 1994.

Peacock, James L. *The Anthropological Lens: Harsh Light, Soft Focus*. Chapel Hill: University of North Carolina Press, 1986.

Peacock, Jeff [pseud.]. Interview by author. Tape recording. Durham, N.C., 12 September 1995.

Peter, Thomas J., and Robert H. Waterman Jr. *In Search of Excellence: Lessons from America's Best-Run Companies*. New York: Warner Books, 1982.

Petrella, Vincent [pseud.]. Interview by author. Tape recording. Durham, N.C., 5 October 1995.

Pettis, John [pseud.]. Questionnaire by author. Durham, N.C., 10 October 1993.

Pollack, Brad [pseud.]. Interview by author. Tape recording. Durham, N.C., 12 July 1991.

Porter, Paul [pseud.]. Interview by author. Tape recording. Durham, N.C., 1 November 2000.

Pratto, Sam [pseud.]. Questionnaire by author. Greensboro, N.C., 14 January 2000.

Raddin, Suzan [pseud.]. Interview by author. Tape recording. Durham, N.C., 20 February 1992.

Raelin, Joseph A. *The Clash of Cultures: Managers Managing Professionals*. Boston: Harvard Business School Press, 1985.

Ramsey, David [pseud.]. Interview by author. Tape recording. Durham, N.C., 5 May 1993.

Raship, Amy. *Food, Eating, and Appetite: Three Case Studies*. Ph.D. diss., University of Pennsylvania, 1987.

Rennard, Carol, and Paul Rennard [pseud.]. Interview by author. Tape recording. Durham, N.C., 24 September 1990.

Reeves, Karen [pseud.]. Interview by author. Tape recording. Durham, N.C., 24 May 1992.

Robinson, John A. "Personal Narratives Reconsidered," *Journal of American Folklore* 94 (1981): 58–85.

Rosati. Robert, MD. "Rap at the Rice House" presentation, Durham, N.C., 20 February 1992.

Rosen, Lily [pseud.]. Interview by author. Tape recording. Durham, N.C., 13 September 1990.

Rosen, Sadie [pseud.]. Interview by author. Tape recording. Durham, N.C., 12 January 1992.

Rosen, Majorie, Marian Etimiades, Sabrina McFarland, Lorenzo Benet,

Todd Gold, Kirstina Johnson, and Lyndon Stambler. "A Terrible Hunger," *People*. 17 February 1992: 92–98.

Ross, John Munder. *The Male Paradox*. New York: Simon & Schuster, 1992.

Roth, Geneen. *Feeding the Hungry Heart: The Experience of Compulsive Overeating*. Bergenfield, N.J.: New American Library, 1982.

Roth, Geneen. *Breaking Free from Compulsive Eating*. Indianapolis: Bobbs-Merrill, 1984.

Roth, Geneen. *When Food Is Love: Exploring the Relationship Between Eating and Intimacy*. New York: Penguin Books, 1992.

Rubenstein, Carin. "Self-Discovery: New Woman's Report on Self-Esteem," *New Woman*. October 1992: 58–62.

Rukenbrod, Fran. "The Role of Support in Changing Eating Habits," *Inside Track/Duke Center for Living*. Fall 1992: 6.

Russo, Jenefer. "Health Risk of Obesity Grossly Overestimated." *Grace-Full Eating Newsletter*. Summer 1992: 4.

Santino, Jack. "Characteristics of Occupational Narratives." In: *Working Americans: Contemporary Approaches to Occupational Folklife,* edited by Robert Byington, 57–70. Los Angeles: California Folklore Society, 1978.

Sarafina, Angelina [pseud.]. Interview by author. Tape recording. Durham, N.C., 10 October, 1992.

Schultz, Olive [pseud.]. Interview by author. Tape recording. Durham, N.C., 10 October 1990.

Schwartz, Felice N. *Breaking with Tradition*. New York: Warner Books, 1992.

Schwartz, H. *Never Satisfied: A Cultural History of Diets, Fantasy, and Fat*. New York: Free Press, 1986.

Sears Catalog. Fall/Winter Annual 93 (1992): 178.

Seid, Roberta Pollack. *Never Too Thin: Why Women Are at War with Their Bodies*. New York: Prentice Hall Press, 1989.

Seldors, Debra [pseud.]. Interview by author. Tape recording. Durham, N.C., 30 January 1991.

Shaw, Kendra [pseud.]. Interview by author. Tape recording. Durham, N.C., 3 August 1993.

Sherrill, Bonnie [pseud.]. Interview by author. Tape recording. Durham, N.C., 4 November 1991.

Sherrill, Martha. "Breast Him-plants: The Joys of Pecs," *Washington Post*. 1 March 1992: F1, F6.

Shamblin, Gwen. *Rise Above: God Can Set You free From Your Weight Problems Forever*. Nashville, Tenn.: Thomas Nelson Publishers, 2000.

Shamblin, Gwen. *The Weigh Down Diet: Inspirational Way to Lose Weight, Stay Slim and Find a New You.* New York: Doubleday.

Shuman, Amy. "The Rhetoric of Portions—All About Eating," *Western Folklore* 30 (1981): 72–80.

Sitco, Cindy [pseud.]. Interview by author. Tape recording. Durham, N.C., 15 June 1995.

Sizemore, Jack [pseud.]. Interview by author. Tape recording. Durham, N.C., 7 June 1991.

Slossberg, Sylvia [pseud.]. Interview by author. Tape recording. Durham, N.C., 15 May 1990.

Snider, Burr. "Fat City," *Esquire*. March 1973: 112–182.

Spiegel Catalog. Fall/Winter 1992: 170.

Stahl, Sandra. *Literary Folkloristics and the Personal Narrative*. Bloomington: Indiana University Press, 1989.

Stahl, Sandra. "The Personal Narrative as Folklore," *Journal of the Folklore Institute* 14 (1977): 9–30.

Standhoff, Sally [pseud.]. Interview by author. Tape recording. Durham, N.C., 2 March 1992.

Stead, Eugene A., MD. "Walter Kempner: A Perspective," *Archives of Internal Medicine* 133 (1974): 756–757.

Steinem, Gloria. "I'm Not the Woman in my Mind," *Parade Magazine* 4 January 1992a: 10–11.

Steinem, Gloria. *Revolution from Within: A Book About Self-Esteem*. Boston: Little, Brown, 1992b.

Steinem, Gloria. *Outrageous Acts and Everyday Rebellions*. New York: Rinehart & Winston, 1983.

Stokes, Richard [pseud.]. Questionnaire by author. Durham, N.C., 15 February 1993.

Structure House Information Folder. Durham, N.C.: Structure House, 1992.

Szekeley, Eva. *Never Too Thin*. Toronto: Women's Press, 1988.

Sutton, Brett. "In the Good Old Way: Primitive Baptist Tradition in an Age of Change." In: *Arts in Earnest: North Carolina Folklife,* edited by Daniel Patterson and Charles G. Zug III. Durham, N.C.: Duke University Press, 1990: 195–215.

Swain, Perry [pseud.]. Interview by author. Tape recording. Durham, N.C., 6 August 1993.

Tannen, Mary. Why the Knife? *Allure*. October 1992: 88–90.

Talley, Jack. Questionnaire by the author. Durham, N.C., 4 November 1999.

Taylor, John Kennedy. *Reclaiming the Mainstream: Individual Feminism Discovered.* Buffalo, N.Y.: Prometheus Books, 1992.

Thompson, Meredith [pseud.]. Interview by author. Tape recording. Durham, N.C., 25 March 1992.

Titon, Jeff Tod. "The Life Story," *Journal of American Folklore* 109 (1980): 276–292.

Trehune, Stephen [pseud.]. Questionnaire by author. Durham, N.C., 5 November 1999.

Tucker, Susan [pseud.]. Interview by author. Tape recording. Durham, N.C., 19 May 1993.

Turner, Victor. *The Drums of Affliction: A Study of Religious Processes Among the Ndembu of Zambia.* Oxford: Claredon Press and the International African Institute, 1968.

UNICE: Stages of Starvation. "Body and Mind," *Durham Herald-Sun.* 4 October 1992: G2.

Van Dijk, Teun A. "Action, Action Description, and Narrative," *New Literary History* 6 (1975): 273–294.

Van Genep, Arnold. *Rites of Passage.* Translated by Monika B. Vizedom and Gabrielle Caffee. Chicago: University of Chicago Press, 1960.

Waldrop, Heidi. *Showing Up for Life: A Recovering Overeater's Triumph Over Compulsion.* Center City, Minn.: Hazelton Educational Materials, 1990.

Ward, Sharon [pseud.]. Interview by author. Tape recording. Durham, N.C., 14 April 1992.

Williams, Julie [pseud.]. Interview by author. Tape recording. Durham, N.C., 7 October 1991.

Williams, Laura. "Fat City," *Aeolos/Duke Chronicle.* 29 March 1978: 4.

Wise, Jim. "Kempner Made Durham, Rice Diet Synonymous," *The Herald Sun.* 12 Oct 1999: 12–14.

Witherspoon, Carol [pseud.]. Interview by author. Tape recording. Durham, N.C., 7 July 1990.

Wolf, Naomi. *The Beauty Myth: How Images of Beauty are Used Against Women.* New York: William Morrow, 1991.

Wolk, Harriet [pseud.]. Interview by author. Tape recording. Durham, N.C., 1 May 1993.

Woodman, Marion, Kae Danson, Mary Hamilton, and Rita Greer Allen. *Leaving My Father's House: A Journey to Conscious Femininity.* Boston: Shambhala, 1992.

glossary

Note: All entries in this glossary came from dieters, hairdressers, shopkeepers, bartenders, and the author's personal experiences, as well as the following articles: Goldstein (1984) and Snider (1973).

Adonis	A young man who loses ten pounds.
Auto-cannibal	A Ricer who is losing weight, i.e., burning his own bacon.
Backsliding	Cheating on the Diet.
Barracuda	The thinnest woman in the Rice House, who is there looking for a husband.
Behemoth	Someone who weighs at least three hundred pounds.
Blubbermaids	Palm Beach matrons.
Body Mass Index (BMI)	Weight in kilograms divided by the square of height in meters. The range of BMI that is now considered normal is around 20 to 24 percent for women and less for men.
Buff and shine	A dieter who has great body potential. All that is needed is a buff and shine (just like a car).
Burned-out bakery boys	Dieters who hang out at the Ninth Street Bakery (now Elmo's), or other coffee shops in Durham, but are not on any diet program.
Cardiac Hill	The inclined Ricer walk on Trinity Avenue. It begins at Duke Street and continues until Mangum Street.

Century Club	The board at the Rice House that displays the names of recent dieters who have lost one hundred pounds or more.
Cherry popped	When a Ricer receives red circles for the first time, indicating extremely low sodium levels.
Chubby chaser	A man (usually) who pursues fat women.
Cooking your own bacon	Losing weight. At this point in the Rice Diet, lipid counts rise because fat cells are digesting themselves.
Crisco Disco	Dieters' Night at the Hilton, where dieters from all programs in Durham went to dance. The term refers to the amount of lard present.
Dead letter	The letter each Ricer receives from the Kempner Clinic concerning the results of medical tests. The letter says the same thing to all Ricers: if one does not reach goal wieght, then one will die a horrible death.
Fat head	Someone with a slim body who thinks like a fat person. A dieter may lose a large amount of weight but still think and act as he or she did when fat.
FFH	Fat Fag Hags. Older, large women dieters who hang around young gay guys in Durham.
Flab flight	Planes that come to the Raleigh-Durham airport from New York, New Jersey, or Florida carrying dieters to Durham.
Five Hundred Club	People who weigh at least five hundred pounds.
Getting lost	Coming to Durham to diet without completing any program.
Gorilla	A very large, unattractive dieter.
Grit	A local townsperson; a native of Durham.
Jumbo	A large young man.
Jumboette	A large young woman.
Last Supper	The last meal consumed before beginning the Rice Diet.
Lean Times	A now-defunct newspaper of the Ricer community.
Lifer	Someone who comes to Durham as a dieter and stays.

Local motion	A young, residential, nondieter lover of a temporary dieter in Durham.
Morbidly obese	Being at least one hundred pounds over one's ideal body weight.
Nickel	A five-hundred-pound woman.
Nylon Bob	A middle-aged man who thinks he's a stud. The term refers to the very tight running shorts often worn by such men.
Obese	Being at least thirty pounds or more over one's ideal body weight.
Off service	Eating illegally at the Rice House when the doctors aren't on the property without paying the medical fees.
Peeling a layer	Losing a significant amount of weight.
Pudged	Water gain caused by premenstrual syndrome.
Pulling the apron	Having sex. After one loses a large amount of weight the skin of the abdomen (the apron) sags and must be lifted in order to have sex.
Ricer	Someone on the Rice Diet.
Ricerhead	The state of dizziness and forgetfulness that occurs when a dieter gets low sodium and potassium levels.
Rotund Ricer	An underground newspaper of the 1970s for the Ricer community.
Saint	Someone who follows the Diet successfully.
Sin City	Concentrations of strip malls and fast-food restaurants that provide tempting opportunities to eat off the Rice Diet, to sin.
Structured	Following the Diet to the letter; planned eating as opposed to unstructured (unplanned and off-limits) eating.
Snowballing	When a Ricer does not lose the necessary amount of weight required, then goes back home, gains even more weight, and returns to Durham fatter than ever.
Spiraling	Going from one diet program to another.
Studly	A really cute young man with the potential for a great body.
Thirteenth Step	The unwritten step of the twelve-step program: Thou shalt not have sex with another dieter.

Thompson Tour	Having plastic surgery to tighten loose skin; Dr. Thompson was a local plastic surgeon who used to do overhauls on many dieters. Now it's Dr. Lanier.
Tit for tat	Men who find physical comfort in a woman larger than they are.
Virgin	A beginning dieter.
Walk-in	A local dieter.
Walking the Wall	Walking around the stone wall that surrounds Duke's east campus, a distance of approximately two miles. Ricers walk the wall religiously. Old Ricers walk it occasionally for old times' sake.
Whale Watch	The pool at Duke Towers Apartments.
Working it	Following the Diet and losing weight rapidly.

About the Author

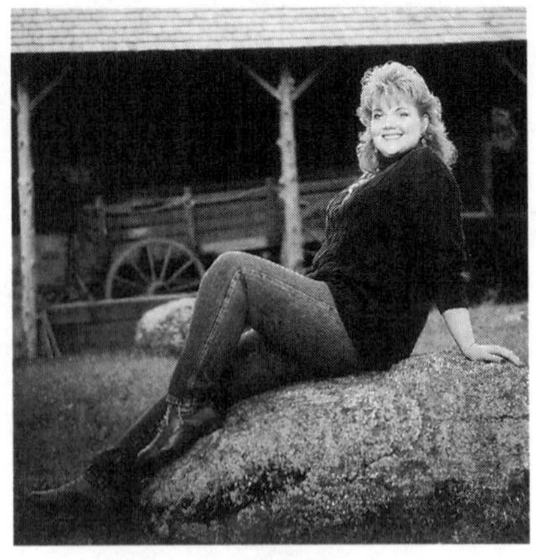

Jean Renfro Anspaugh began collecting dieting stories in 1989 as part of a master's class project in personal narrative. The tales she collected revealed to her a diet culture, complete with values, aesthetics, work ethic, religious ethos, and language all its own. Her collection became the foundation of her master's thesis, and she received her M.A. in Folklore from the University of North Carolina, Chapel Hill in 1993. At first, professionals in her field rejected her work, saying in so many words, "Who cares about fat folks?" However, Jean has now proven her case for a separate diet culture and has earned a reputation as the Folklorist of the Fat.

Professionally she is interested in the products of diet culture: the stories, the tales and the behavior of dieters. Personally she has been a dieter all her life. She lost one hundred pounds on the Rice Diet, gained half of it back, took some of it off again, and still zigzags up and down the scale. Yet, something extraordinary happened to her on the road to thinness. She stopped defining herself by others' expectations of her. She also realized that she was not alone. Through her professional work, she discovered that there are thousands of people just like her who have struggled all of their lives with the central, defining factor of their lives—obesity. It was a transforming moment in her life to recognize that she was part of a culture. That recognition has helped her transcend fat identity, so that she could get on with her life without reference to her weight.

When she is not out collecting more stories, she is a wife and mother. She enjoys living her life no longer limited by her body type. She hopes that her collection of stories can help others achieve their own transformations and find satisfaction in their lives, no matter what the scale, society, or concerned family members say.

Fat Like Us is her first book.